Contents

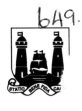

EVERYTHING

YOU NEED TO KNOW ABOUT...

Breastfeeding

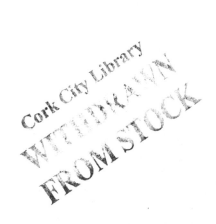

EVERYTHING

YOU NEED TO KNOW ABOUT...

Breastfeeding

SUZANNE FREDREGILL

AND RAY FREDREGILL

David & Charles

A DAVID & CHARLES BOOK

David & Charles is a subsidiary of F+W (UK) Ltd.,

an F+W Publications Inc. company

First published in the UK in 2004

First published in the USA as The Everything® Breastfeeding Book,

by Adams Media Corporation in 2002

Project Manager Ian Kearey

Cover Design Ali Myer

A catalogue record for this book is available from the British Library.

ISBN 0 7153 2065 3

Printed in Great Britain by CPI Bath

for David & Charles

Brunel House   Newton Abbot   Devon

Visit our website at www.davidandcharles.co.uk

David & Charles books are available from all good bookshops;

alternatively you can contact our Orderline on (0)1626 334555 or

write to us at FREEPOST EX2110, David & Charles Direct,

Newton Abbot, TQ12 4ZZ (no stamp required UK mainland).

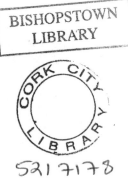

Dedication

To our breastfed children, Meaghan and Ian, and to our parents.

Introduction

Making a 'decision' to breastfeed is really very new. Since long before recorded history, breastfeeding was the only choice women had. If a mother was unable to nurse her child, family or friends who were lactating would nurse the baby for her. In some cases, wet nurses were employed by the wealthy – a wet nurse was a lactating woman who was paid to nurse and care for another's child, and who often nursed her young charges in addition to her own children.

Today, about two-thirds of UK mothers begin breastfeeding their babies, but although breastfeeding is enthusiastically endorsed by health professionals, many women still give up breastfeeding in the first few weeks. Contrary to many myths, most women can breastfeed their babies, given the right support and information. Your breastfeeding relationship with your child will have far-reaching rewards for you, your baby and your entire family.

Nursing might be one of the most satisfying relationships you've ever had. There's nothing like the emotional closeness of breastfeeding. When your baby looks up at you adoringly and smiles, you'll know you've made the right choice.

Breastfed children have fewer infections, fewer digestive problems and better brain development than formula-fed babies, and that's just the beginning. Breastfeeding also helps your body recover from labour and birth, and decreases your risk of pre-menopausal breast cancer. Women who breastfeed have a lower risk of developing ovarian cancer and broken bones due to osteoporosis in later life. There are even financial and environmental advantages. Breastfeeding your child is a responsible, loving and natural choice.

However, although breastfeeding is natural, learning this new skill doesn't come naturally to everyone. Some women are lucky enough to experience only a few problems, but many need a little help at first. In the past, women grew up surrounded by breastfeeding friends and family members. Girls growing up then had the opportunity to learn the 'womanly art' from their female role models. By the time they had children, they had seen and perhaps assisted with breastfeeding on many occasions. If they had a problem, they could consult their mothers, female friends or a midwife.

Things changed in the 20th century. Bottle feeding of infant formulas became much more common than breastfeeding. Women were persuaded by both advertisers and the medical community that infant formula was at least as good as breastmilk, and certainly more convenient. Today, we know that nothing compares to breastmilk. Unfortunately, decades of bottle feeding have left most women without the social support and knowledge necessary for breastfeeding success, and now we have to rely on a more formal method of breastfeeding education.

This book will provide you with techniques, tips and insights that will enhance your breastfeeding experience. The information provided is based on current research and recommended best practices in the field of breastfeeding education.

You *can* breastfeed. There is no better nourishment for your baby than your own milk, which is specially designed for your child, whether premature or full term, infant or toddler. With a little preparation, practice, confidence and patience, you'll be well on your way towards breastfeeding success.

CHAPTER 1

The Importance of Breastfeeding

Despite all the fantastic things humans have accomplished, we've never been able to come up with a better food than breastmilk for your baby. That's not to say we haven't tried – the formula options available can be mind-boggling. Luckily for us, the simplest choice is also the healthiest choice; no infant formula can meet your baby's needs the way your own breastmilk does.

Breastfeeding Is Good for Your Baby

Breastmilk is the elixir of life for your baby. Each precious drop gives her exactly what she needs in just the right amounts. It's an incredible mixture that's constantly changing to meet your baby's needs.

Digestibility

One of the greatest advantages of breastmilk is how easily your baby can digest it. This is especially important during the first year of life, when your baby will be growing more rapidly than at any other time. Part of the reason breastmilk is so digestible is that the proteins are smaller than formula proteins. The vitamins and minerals in breastmilk are also more easily absorbed by your baby's body than those found in formula or other supplements. But breastmilk goes beyond just being easy to digest.

Breastmilk is the best milk for your baby – and it's not just this book that says so! Internationally, the World Health Organization, the United Nations Children's Fund (UNICEF), the International Confederation of Midwives and the International Federation of Gynaecology and Obstetrics, and specifically in Britain the Department of Health, the Natural Childbirth Trust (NCT) and the Royal College of Midwives all recommend exclusive breastfeeding for at least the first six months of your baby's life.

Enzymes in breastmilk work with your baby's digestive system to help her get the most out of every feeding. As a result, breastmilk goes through your baby's system twice as fast as formula, at the same time providing her with better nourishment than any other food source.

Yes, this means that your young, breastfed baby will have more frequent bowel movements than formula-fed babies of the same age. It also means your nursing baby will want to eat more frequently than a formula-fed baby. But your baby will spit up less and have fewer cases of indigestion. Because breastfed infants generally eat smaller meals than formula-fed babies, there's less opportunity for spitting up (possetting).

The easy digestibility of breastmilk is also important in lessening the severity of gastro-oesophageal reflux (GER). This is a heartburn-like pain that happens when stomach acids back up into your baby's oesophagus. A circular muscle where the esophagus meets the stomach normally prevents this from occurring; however, in some babies it takes most of their first year of life for that muscle to develop properly.

If you've ever had acid reflux or heartburn, just imagine having it as a baby. As the old Lesley Gore song, 'It's My Party', says, 'You would cry, too, if it happened to you!'

Stools

As a direct result of breastmilk's digestibility, your baby's stools will be smaller, softer and less likely to knock you out. No one is promising that changing nappies will be like a trip to the perfume counter, but with fewer fats and proteins passing through your baby's system undigested, the smell of stools is not just reduced, it's changed.

tips

Keeping an eye on your baby's nappies is a good way to assess your milk production. Babies typically have at least eight to ten wet nappies and four to six stools per day when they are getting enough to eat.

Immunity

At birth and until approximately four months of age, your child's immune system is underdeveloped. All sorts of viruses, fungi, bacteria and other villains will try to invade your baby's body. Without a mature immune system, she's an easy target for them, but, once again, it's breastmilk to the rescue!

Many of the ingredients in your breastmilk help fight infections or promote the growing strength of your baby's own immune system. Breastmilk contains ingredients that shield the intestines, help friendly bacteria grow, keep necessary iron away from the invading cells, and cut through the invaders' cell walls.

An exciting study on breastmilk and immunology was featured in the June 1999 issue of the American *Discover* magazine under the title 'Got Cancer Killers?' A protein (dubbed 'HAMLET') in breastmilk causes cancer cells to commit suicide. HAMLET is reported to be deadly to 'every cancer we test it against', say the researchers. Imagine if a cancer cure has been literally under our noses all along!

Perhaps most amazingly, breastmilk is a living substance. Like blood, it's teeming with millions of disease-fighting cells called antibodies. These antibodies are nature's way of immunizing your baby against every disease you have ever been exposed to. And that protection constantly improves. If you are exposed to a new germ, your body will pass on immunity to that germ to your baby through your milk. 'Breastmilk immunization' can happen before you even notice the first symptoms of illness.

Adults who were breastfed as infants have lower incidences of diabetes, Crohn's disease and coronary heart disease. Furthermore, research has established that breastmilk kills germs in babies' mouths and helps heal mothers' cracked nipples. Some mums even put it on cuts and scrapes. It's like your immune system in an easy-to-use liquid.

Intelligence

Your baby's brain grows at a fantastic rate in the first few months. You won't always be able to tell as she lies in your arms looking so serene, but this is her brain's busiest developmental stage. Behind that cute brow, there's a firestorm of activity: neural pathways are forming, and with every moment, some paths are strengthened and others fade. Your baby needs the proper materials for this important work, and your breastmilk is a virtual shopping list of exactly those ingredients. Studies have found up to a 10-point IQ advantage for breastfed children over those fed on formula milk.

Fats and sugars in your milk are custom-engineered for brain growth. Babies need fat for brain development for at least the first two years of their lives. The fats found in your breastmilk help form the insulation on the electrical wiring of your baby's brain, and they can also make your baby more able, too.

Your milk is specially made for your baby, just as cow's milk is made for calves and goat's milk is made for kids. The types of proteins, fats and other nutrients found in cow's milk are just what a baby cow needs, but your baby's needs are different. Your breastmilk will actually change as your baby grows – for example, your body produces less fat for older babies than for newborns, while premature infants receive breastmilk that's richer and higher in calories.

Colic

Colicky babies cry and make a lot of fuss – it's impossible to over-emphasize just how much; it seems like an unending stomach ache. While the exact causes are unknown, one thing remains true in every single case: babies with colic are unhappy. Mothers with colicky babies aren't exactly thrilled about colic, either.

The good news is that babies who are exclusively breastfed have a much lower incidence of colic (although that's not to say it can't and doesn't happen). Breastfeeding infants can be colicky, and a newborn's digestive system might not be able to fully digest anything – even breastmilk. However, when breastfed babies are colicky, the colic is usually less severe and lasts for a shorter period of time than it would be if they were fed on formula.

Emotional State

Babies often fall asleep at the breast, full and content. Breastmilk contains ingredients that stimulate your baby's body to produce a hormone called cholecystokinin (CCK). CCK relaxes your baby and helps her sleep, as it's the same hormone that makes you feel drowsy after a big meal.

The act of nursing is also comforting to your baby and satisfies her need to suck. The skin-to-skin contact keeps her warm. Your body temperature will actually adjust itself in response to hers. Nestled in your arms, she feels safe and secure. The closeness and intimacy of the feeding experience fosters your baby's sense of trust and makes it easier for her to communicate her needs to you. And you smell good to your baby, just like your milk.

The profound emotional connection you make with your baby grows into the connection you will have with your child. Nursing your baby makes you more in tune with her needs and feelings. She will feel secure and develop a trust in you that will serve as a strong foundation for her entire childhood.

Weight

Breastfed babies generally don't gain weight as quickly in the first few days as formula-fed babies, but they soon catch up. Many breastfeeding mothers worry that they cannot see how much their baby is taking in, but if your baby is gaining weight at a good rate and is producing several wet and dirty nappies each day, the chances are that you have nothing to worry about. If you have any concerns about weight, talk to your doctor or health visitor.

Formula and breastmilk generally average about the same number of calories by volume. The difference is in the other ingredients and in the delivery system, depending on the basis of the formula. For example, cow's milk is made to build body mass. The types of fats and proteins it contains encourage early weight gain. This makes sense for an animal that will gain so much weight in its first year of life. Breastmilk, on the other hand, contains a healthier balance of body and brain builders. It also changes as your baby suckles. At first, your baby gets the protein-rich foremilk. As she continues to nurse, your calorie-rich hindmilk lets down.

Facial Development

Babies suck on breasts in a different way to bottles. The breast fills the mouth more completely and breastfeeding works the entire mouth, while bottle feeding exercises only the front. The sucking movements affect babies' facial development. Breastfed babies tend to have larger nasal space and better jaw alignment, which means a reduced risk of snoring, sleep apnoea and orthodontic work later in life.

Allergies

Allergies are believed to be the cause of many problems in both children and adults, ranging from hay fever and wheat, nut and gluten allergies all the way through to behavioural difficulties. Infants are especially vulnerable to food allergies because of what some doctors call the leaky gut syndrome, in which the cells lining a baby's intestinal walls are just not packed together densely enough at birth to stop food proteins, or allergens, from entering the body.

f@ct

Colostrum is the yellowish fluid your breasts produce immediately following the birth of your baby. Many cultures have regarded colostrum as 'dirty milk' and kept it from babies, but the reality is just the opposite: it's exactly what a newborn needs. Colostrum knocks out germs even more effectively than regular breastmilk and helps your baby get a healthy start in many other ways.

If you practise breastfeeding exclusively during your baby's first six months, you don't need to worry too much about food allergies. If you feed formula, however, you need to be aware of a host of potential allergens in the mix.

Breastmilk meets your baby's needs perfectly. It contains substances that help 'seal the leaks' in your baby's intestinal lining while other substances help the lining to grow. At around six months of age, your baby's leaky intestinal lining achieves 'closure', and babies become less sensitive to allergens and can start to try different foods.

Breastfeeding Is Good for You, Too

Not only is putting your baby to breast good for your baby, it's been shown time and again to have some impressive advantages for mothers as well. By breastfeeding, you will experience short-term benefits such as delayed periods, as well as reduced risks of pre-menopausal breast cancer and osteoporosis in later life.

Postpartum Recovery

You will be encouraged to feed your baby as soon after birth as possible. In addition to the fact that professional childbirth assistants nearly always advocate breastfeeding for babies, it's also an important part of your natural recovery from labour and delivery. Breastfeeding releases the hormone oxytocin, which causes your uterus to contract, thereby helping stop the flow of blood and delivering the placenta in one piece. If you choose not to breastfeed, your doctor will intervene with an injection of Pitocin, a synthetic form of oxytocin, to provide assistance with the delivery of your placenta.

Amenorrhoea

Amenorrhoea is big word with a little definition: no periods. Many women find that they enjoy time off from their menses for the first six months of breastfeeding. The benefits of this little break are more than just convenience.

Lactational amenorrhoea (the pausing of your menstrual cycle while breastfeeding) means reduced fertility. As long as you are exclusively breastfeeding, you're much less likely to become pregnant – however, every woman is different, so it is important to use other methods of contraception as well. Ask your GP or health visitor for advice. Best of all, it's completely natural.

tips

Mother Nature's family planning: six weeks of postpartum abstinence followed by six months of breastfeeding-induced amenorrhoea gives you over 16 months between births. However, amenorrhoea is different for every woman, and sometimes the shortest separation from your baby can derail the process.

The other benefit of lactational amenorrhoea is the prevention of anaemia. Because breastfeeding removes iron from your body at a rate of about 0.3 milligrams per day, doctors have long considered it to be a cause of anaemia in new mothers. As researcher Ted Greiner has pointed out, the amount of iron new mothers would normally lose with their period is retained when their menses stop due to breastfeeding. In other words, instead of losing large amounts of iron during your period, you can lose much smaller amounts to your baby.

Traditionally, people have viewed breastfeeding as being a 'strain' on the mother's body. But today we know that this is not the case at all. In fact, breastfeeding can play an important role in helping mothers recover from pregnancy and childbirth. Ample evidence exists that pregnancy can cause maternal anaemia; through breastfeeding, nature provides the remedy.

Cancer Prevention

You'll enjoy a significant reduction in your risk for breast cancer as a result of nursing your child. This protection has been found in women who have breastfed for as little as three months. The longer you nurse, the lower your risk of developing breast cancer. If you breastfeed for two years, you may cut your chances of developing breast cancer by a significant amount.

Other cancers are less likely in women who have breastfed, too. Ovarian, uterine and cervical cancers are less common in women who have breastfed. No one is entirely certain how breastfeeding protects you from these potential killers, but one theory suggests that lactation's suppression of oestrogen production plays an important role. Oestrogen is a hormone that promotes cell growth in your reproductive anatomy and has been linked with female reproductive cancers. When you lactate, your body produces less oestrogen. Lower levels of oestrogen mean less growth, which in turn provides less opportunity for cancers to develop.

Osteoporosis

You might have heard that pregnancy and breastfeeding deplete your body of calcium, leading to an increased risk of osteoporosis (brittle bones). The first part of that statement is true. Pregnancy and breastfeeding do use up your body's calcium reserve, but breastfeeding can actually help prevent osteoporosis. Here's how it works.

Weaning stimulates your body to increase bone density. Your postlactation bones will be stronger than they would have been if you had never breastfed at all. All you need to do is get enough calcium in your diet, and your body takes care of the rest. Broccoli, almonds, wholemeal bread, oranges, peanut butter, dairy products and beans are all calcium-rich foods.

Weight Loss

How would you like to eat more and still lose weight? When you breastfeed, your body will burn up the fat it stored during pregnancy to make milk. In addition, breastfeeding will encourage your uterus to return to its pre-pregnancy size, helping you to get back into shape all over your body.

Bonding

Nursing your little bundle of joy puts her close to you and gives you the chance to coo, cuddle and take her in with all of your senses. We all talk about connecting with our children, and with breastfeeding the connection is real and physical. Skin-to-skin contact and suckling release powerful stress-reducing hormones (oxytocin and prolactin) in your body that relax you and give you a calm, pleasurable feeling. Those same hormones help you to literally fall in love with your newborn. Prolactin is sometimes called the 'mothering hormone' because of the way it intensifies nurturing behaviour.

If the 'baby blues' extend beyond the first two weeks following the birth of your baby, you may be suffering from postpartum depression. If you find yourself feeling lethargic, develop loss of appetite or have a hard time functioning, contact your doctor or midwife as soon as you can. You're not alone, and support is available.

Prolactin is also a natural tranquillizer. Within minutes of latching on, you might begin to relax so much that you feel yourself getting sleepy. That's one of nature's little rewards.

These same hormones also prevent the short-term feeling of sadness that some women experience after childbirth. The 'baby blues' are a result of the sudden drop in pregnancy hormones in your body after delivery. The baby blues can delay the bonding process and leave you unable to enjoy the first few days of motherhood. Breastfeeding signals to your body to release the hormones that prevent those blues. If you breastfeed immediately following birth and wean gradually at a time of your choice, you may be able to avoid the baby blues altogether.

Satisfaction

Breastfeeding can give you a strong sense of accomplishment, pride and continuity with life and the world. You don't have to be an Earth Mother to appreciate the spiritual side of childbearing or your body's ability to feed your baby. Nursing is a powerful aspect of motherhood. Trusting your body to nourish your child is a deeply satisfying experience, and breastfeeding is a truly wonderful privilege.

Breastfeeding's Other Benefits

So, breastfeeding is good for your baby and good for you. And in case that isn't enough to sell you on the idea, consider the secondary effects of going *au naturel*: no recycling, no late-night trips to the 24-hour shop – and, best of all, breastmilk is free!

Environmental Convenience

Breastmilk isn't made in a factory or transported to your local supermarket. No chemicals are used to manufacture colourful labels. You don't usually need a non-biodegradable bottle or processed petrochemical teat to use it. When you've finished feeding, you don't have anything left over to be taken to the landfill site. Maybe breastfeeding won't save the world all on its own, but then again, every little bit helps – after all, this is the world we'll be leaving to our children.

Formula needs to be prepared and heated. Those few extra seconds can seem like an eternity when your hungry baby is crying – especially in the middle of the night. With nursing, you don't have to worry about the quality of the water or the temperature of the milk. Breastmilk is the original convenience food.

Penny Wise

Breastfeeding will also save you a significant amount of money when compared with feeding infant formula. The cost of formula feeding is at least £350–420 per year, depending on your (or your baby's) choice of formula. Then you shell out more cash for the extra bottles, liners and teats, and maybe even for dry cleaning to remove those stubborn formula-spit-up stains.

One of the nicest things about breastfeeding is the convenience. The milk is always the perfect temperature, it's always clean, and you can't forget your breasts when you leave the house!

Just for Dads

There is no reason for new fathers to feel excluded by the feeding process. There is a lot that you can do to get involved and assist your partner, whether you plan to feed your baby expressed milk from a bottle, or just offer the practical and emotional support that is so important for all nursing mothers.

CHAPTER 2

Who Can Breastfeed?

The vast majority of mothers can breastfeed successfully. If you're able to give birth, you're almost certainly able to nurse your baby. There are exceptions, but these are uncommon and usually temporary. Most women who believed they were unable to breastfeed were probably just missing the two most important things every nursing mother really needs – confidence and support.

Breast Issues

The fact is that breast 'issues' are most often a result of preconceived notions. In the past, a lack of information, education and encouragement to breastfeed left many mothers making assumptions about why it wouldn't work for them. With the proper preparation and support, virtually all mothers can provide natural nourishment to their babies.

Breast Size

Breast size is mostly a matter of fat content, not milk-gland content. Small-chested women may actually have an advantage over their bustier friends when nursing low birth weight or premature babies. Very small babies sometimes find it difficult to latch onto an engorged breast. In those cases, smaller breasts can be an advantage.

My nipples are pierced. Will the holes interfere with nursing?
Many women with pierced nipples have successfully breastfed. However, piercing of the nipples sometimes scars the milk ducts and inhibits the flow of milk. If your piercings have been infected or if you have multiple nipple piercings, you may find breastfeeding difficult. All jewellery must be removed before nursing.

If your breasts are large and you're self-conscious about their size, don't let that discourage you from breastfeeding, either. Large breasts don't generally get much larger with lactation. They also tend to leak less than smaller breasts.

There are advantages and disadvantages to different breast sizes, of course, but regardless of your size, stick with it, become informed and stay confident. You can have a successful breastfeeding experience.

Nipples

Just as with breasts, nipples come in a variety of types. There are nipples the size of champagne corks, nipples that hide inside the breast (inverted) and nipples that point up, down or sideways. It's not unusual for a woman to have one nipple that's inverted and another that's not.

No matter what type of nipples you have, breastfeeding is possible. Inverted nipples can be coaxed out and large nipples can be worked around. Other mums have done it, and you can, too.

Adoptive Mums

Yes, you can nurse your adopted baby! The process is not easy, but it can be done and has been done by many women. Your milk production can be started with the help of a breast pump and a little patience. However, initiating lactation without pregnancy requires a serious commitment.

A woman who produces milk for her own baby has the advantage of pregnancy; for nine months, her body has been preparing to feed a baby. Without those pregnancy hormones, you'll have to rely on manual stimulation as explained in detail in Chapter 12.

fact

The initiation of milk production is called 'lactogenesis'. Although there are new hormonal therapies being developed that can help a woman to lactate without pregnancy, these procedures may produce unpleasant side effects as well as the risk of unknown future complications. Check with your doctor.

Adoptive mums don't usually produce enough milk to fully feed a young infant, but don't let that discourage you. Nursing your baby isn't only about nutrition – any amount of milk you produce is a precious gift for your child, and the experience of nursing will be wonderful for both of you.

Drugs and Alcohol

The best practice when you're breastfeeding is to steer clear of street drugs and to limit your alcohol intake. Medical conditions or addictions can stand in the way of a drug-free lactation. If you smoke or drink, you'll need to make some changes during pregnancy and while nursing your child.

Medicine

The two main issues to consider before taking any medicine while breastfeeding are: do the benefits to my health outweigh any risk to my baby; and do I need to wean my child to protect her from this medication? Some medications are harmless to your nursing infant, while others are less safe. Fortunately, permanent weaning is rarely necessary. Although many medicines will enter your milk supply, the amounts that reach your child are usually small. As a result, breastfeeding is compatible with a wide variety of medicines.

Some medications are not safe to use while breastfeeding. If temporary weaning due to medication becomes necessary, it's important to use a breast pump to maintain your milk production. You'll need to 'pump and dump' as often as your baby would nurse.

If you're taking a prescription drug on a doctor's order, remind your doctor that you plan to breastfeed. Some doctors routinely advise mothers to wean while medicated because they are not well informed about breastfeeding. Your midwife or health visitor is also a good source of information.

While many drugs are considered safe for nursing mothers, certain types are considered off-limits. Some of these drugs will affect your baby, while others can decrease your milk production. Some sources consider most medications to be off limits, while other sources consider the majority of medications to be compatible with breastfeeding.

It can be difficult to know whose advice to take. Doctors and drug companies both like to be on the safe side. If they don't have proof that a particular drug is safe for breastfeeding, they recommend weaning. As a rule, you should be able to safely take any medicine your child can take and continue to nurse without worry. However, you should avoid combining medications if possible.

As your baby grows, it becomes safer for you to take medications. In the meantime, take the minimum amount necessary to ensure your comfort and health. An unwell mother has a hard time taking care of her child. Sometimes, you have to take care of yourself first.

Alcohol

While alcohol was advised against during your pregnancy, the rules for lactating mothers are a little more lenient – a glass of wine with dinner or some champagne at a wedding is not completely out of the question. However, you need to be careful.

Alcohol does find its way into your milk. The negative effects for your baby include possible long-term immunity weakness and nervous system disorders. Infants in the first months of life are especially sensitive to alcohol's effects, since their livers are not yet mature enough to eliminate it easily from their bloodstream. Older babies, who rely less on their mother for nursing and who have more body mass, are better able to tolerate small amounts of alcohol in your breastmilk.

The good news is that alcohol clears from your breastmilk at about the same rate it clears from your bloodstream. If you have a single drink immediately after nursing, your milk should be alcohol-free by the time you nurse again in two to three hours (depending on your weight).

If your baby sleeps with you, your use of drugs or alcohol can be deadly. Normally, you sleep lightly when your child shares the bed. Parents 'under the influence' are less aware. There are cases where babies died because a parent who had taken drugs or drunk alcohol rolled over and accidentally suffocated them.

Tradition maintains that an occasional serving of alcohol helps a mother produce more milk. Contrary to folk wisdom, however, alcohol appears to have a negative impact on successful breastfeeding. Studies have demonstrated a change in the taste and smell of breastmilk when mum drinks alcohol, and babies don't generally like it. Alcohol also reduces the levels of prolactin and oxytocin that are produced in your body when your baby suckles. Prolactin aids in milk production as well as emotional bonding, while oxytocin plays a key role in your milk ejection, or letdown, response.

If you drink frequently, you may find your child weaning far earlier than you had planned, as your milk production, delivery and flavour might lead to early weaning. On the other hand, an occasional drink appears to be relatively harmless if you allow it to clear from your bloodstream before nursing.

Smoking

If you haven't given up smoking already, this is a great time to stop. If you're a new parent, there are some important reasons to kick the habit: smoking during pregnancy leads to low birth weight, reduced IQ, heart and lung difficulties for your baby, and an increased risk of complications following birth for both mother and child. After delivery, smoking continues to threaten your child's health.

If you nurse your baby and smoke, nicotine will find its way into your milk. Heavy smokers (more than 20 a day) may find that their babies suffer from intestinal upsets and nervousness. Heavy smokers are also nearly twice as likely as non-smokers to have colicky babies. As with alcohol, smoking has been linked to early weaning due to lowered milk production and inhibited letdown.

Which smoking cessation product is best?
If you would like to stop smoking, discuss your options with your GP or health visitor before using any nicotine replacement therapies such as patches or gum. Always tell the practitioner that you are breastfeeding at the start of the meeting.

Secondhand smoke is far more dangerous to babies than nicotine – everyone needs to keep cigarette smoke far away from babies. Secondhand smoke has been linked to Sudden Infant Death Syndrome (SIDS) and respiratory infections. Just as you would insist on clean hands to hold your baby, insist on clean air for her, too. If Dad smokes, keeping smoke away from the baby is a great way to show he loves her.

The bottom line on smoking and breastfeeding is this: the benefits of breastfeeding generally outweigh the hazards of nicotine in your milk, but not those of secondhand smoke. If you can stop, your whole family wins. If you continue to smoke while nursing, you run a risk. At a minimum, try to cut down and keep the smoke away from your baby.

Controlled Substances

As with other drugs, controlled substances can interfere with your milk supply and letdown reflex. Marijuana, for instance, has been shown to reduce a mother's milk production by decreasing the level of prolactin she produces. It's also important to realize that any drugs you take can end up in your breastmilk, sometimes in a concentrated form. When you use the drugs, your baby uses them too. The damage done to a developing infant can be serious and permanent.

Street drugs such as heroin and cocaine may be cut with harmful chemicals, and you can't be sure about their strength. Most importantly, recreational use of drugs impairs your ability to be a good parent. Many drugs cause a loss of judgment and coordination, while good parenting requires a clear head.

If you have an addiction to a controlled substance, talk to your doctor about getting help.

Herbal Remedies

While it's always important to be careful, many herbs are safe for breastfeeding women. There are herbs that can increase or decrease your milk supply. Others can take the place of regular, over-the-counter medications. If you choose to use herbal products, follow these guidelines:

❑ Check with your doctor.
❑ Use a brand that lists all active ingredients. The fewer ingredients, the better.
❑ Stick with a reputable brand.

❏ Check the expiry date.
❏ Bear in mind that herbal tinctures contain alcohol.

Herbs may seem natural and safe, but they are potent pharmacological substances. Many of the medicines found at the pharmacy are derived from herbs. Always discuss remedies with your GP or health visitor.

Multiple Births

Two babies? Now you know why you have two breasts! You can nurse twins or even triplets without worrying about your milk supply. Your breasts are marvellous self-regulating milk production centres. The amount of milk they make is directly related to the amount of milk removed by a baby's suckling – more suckling equals more milk.

Caesarean Section

If you've delivered your child by Caesarean section, breastfeeding will help you to regain trust in your body's ability to mother while helping you to bond with your new baby. Sometimes, women who have delivered by Caesarean feel disappointed that their bodies have somehow failed them, but breastfeeding reinforces your confidence in your body's ability to nourish and nurture the new life you have brought into the world.

Although a Caesarean is major surgery and your incision can be tender, your baby can nurse without causing stress on your sutures.

Mother's Medical Conditions

You may have a chronic health concern or condition, but this should not necessarily prevent you from breastfeeding successfully. Your health-care providers can give you information on the best way to accommodate your situation while providing the best feeding option for your baby.

Diabetes

Many diabetic women have successfully breastfed their children. You'll need to pay close attention to your diet because lactating can seriously affect your blood glucose levels. Keep lots of water and snacks handy when nursing to help you avoid becoming hypoglycaemic. Your regular insulin injections are safe for your nursing child. Discuss your medication options with your doctor.

Diabetes will present you with some special challenges. Diabetic mothers tend to get more yeast infections and suffer from mastitis more than non-diabetics. You'll need to give extra attention to your breasts and watch out for plugged milk ducts.

You're giving your baby a wonderful gift when you nurse. Best of all, breastfeeding your baby will help her to avoid becoming diabetic, too – studies show that breastfed babies have a lowered incidence of Type 1 diabetes as well as fewer occurrences of obesity as adults.

HIV

In the UK, HIV-positive women are advised not to breastfeed because the risk of infecting your baby through your milk is so great. Although in some countries women are told to breastfeed babies who are HIV-positive, remember that babies are born with their mother's antibodies, so it is not possible to confirm a baby's HIV status until he is at least 10 months old.

If you feel strongly that you do want to breastfeed, seek advice from your GP and midwife before the birth, and be aware that by breastfeeding your baby without seeking advice you may be risking legal intervention. Organizations such as the Terrence Higgins Trust (*www.tht.org.uk*, tel 0845 122 1200) can provide help and support.

Herpes

Herpes can be deadly to newborns if a mother contracts it during the last trimester of pregnancy. If you become infected at that time, a Caesarean might be your only option. Herpes on a woman's breast is less of a threat. With a few precautions, you can safely nurse your baby.

If you develop a herpes sore on your nipple, it's best not to let your baby nurse from that side until it's healed. Use a pump on the affected breast to maintain your milk supply. If the sore is somewhere else on your breast, cover it with a bandage or pad and continue to nurse as usual. Any time you have an active outbreak of herpes, whether genital or oral (cold sores), you should take extra precautions. Wash your hands before handling your baby or your breasts, and always keep your child away from herpes sores.

Cancer

A diagnosis of cancer doesn't mean it's time to wean – babies cannot develop cancer through breastmilk, and many cancer treatments are compatible with breastfeeding. If you are determined, you can continue to nurse your child despite biopsies or even more involved surgeries. However, there are some treatments that can affect your ability to breastfeed. With any type of cancer, it's important that you discuss your desire to breastfeed with your doctor and follow her advice.

 Tuberculosis is usually spread by adults with active TB, and children under the age of five have the greatest risk of infection. Mothers with untreated, active tuberculosis should not breastfeed their babies.

If your cancer treatment involves chemotherapy or the injection of radioactive compounds, you must wean your baby until those substances have left your body, as some radioactive agents remain in your body for many months.

Chemotherapy drugs are among the most toxic medicines used. They will enter your breastmilk, and even a tiny amount can be harmful to your child. If you plan to resume nursing, you should 'pump and dump' your milk until your doctor gives you the all-clear to nurse.

Breast Surgeries

If you've had breast surgery, talk to your doctor about the possibility of breastfeeding your child. You might be pleasantly surprised. If it turns out that you are unable to produce enough milk for exclusive breastfeeding, don't be discouraged. Whatever amount of milk you can produce for your baby is wonderful, as every little bit contains the antibodies and nutrients that only you can provide. Remember, too, that nursing your baby isn't only about the milk – breastfeeding is a special and loving time with your baby.

If you want to nurse your child, you can purchase one of a number of supplemental feeding systems. These devices allow your baby to nurse from your breast while receiving formula through tiny tubes. Another choice is to simply bottle feed formula after each nursing session.

Breast Reduction

Most women who have had breast reduction surgery can still produce some milk. However, this type of surgery typically leaves women unable to produce enough milk to exclusively nurse their babies. In some reductions, the nipple is completely removed from the breast and reattached in a new location. If the nipples were completely severed and are numb as a consequence, breastfeeding is not possible. In some rare cases, severed nerves have actually grown back after breast reduction surgery, but this is very unusual.

Breast Augmentation

Breast augmentation surgery will not usually interfere with a woman's ability to produce milk. Most surgeons make the incisions near the armpit or under the fold of the breast. With the nipple left undisturbed, nursing is generally unaffected. Some new mothers worry about implant leakage into their milk supply, but there's no need to let that bother you – the horror stories about leaking implants that were widely reported in the news a few years ago have turned out to be unsupported by any valid research. Whether your implants are silicone or saline, your milk is safe for your baby.

Baby's Medical Conditions

Although you may be in excellent health, it is possible that one of several infant conditions will present challenges for your breastfeeding plans. While hospitals routinely screen newborns for a large number of disorders, it is important that you notify your doctor if you have a family history of galactosaemia, PKU or any other hereditary conditions. A hospital lactation consultant may be available to guide you through these and other situations.

Jaundice

Jaundice is a condition that affects many newborns to a greater or lesser extent. Jaundiced babies appear yellow or orange because of an excess of bilirubin, a substance produced when a baby's body breaks down surplus red blood cells. Jaundiced babies are often sleepy and need to be woken up to nurse. Normal newborn jaundice occurs within the first week of life and lasts no more than two weeks. Other types of jaundice may be due to medical conditions that require more advanced treatment.

If your baby is jaundiced, nursing will help. Bilirubin leaves your child's body through his stools. Frequent nursings at the breast help your baby have frequent stools and eliminate excess bilirubin quickly.

Premature Birth

Premature babies have special needs: they are usually very small and more susceptible to infections, and they suckle less effectively than full-term babies. To complicate breastfeeding even further, premature babies might need to be placed in a Neonatal Intensive Care Unit (NICU). With IVs and other medical procedures, nursing might not be possible.

Many parents feel helpless when their baby needs so much medical attention, but only a mother can provide her baby with the perfect food. Your breastmilk is exactly formulated for your child, whether the baby is premature or full term. Refer to Chapter 7 for alternative feeding methods. Pumping will help you feel connected with your child, even when you're unable to hold her; it will also keep your milk supply up for the day she's able to nurse.

Galactosaemia

Galactosaemia is a rare, inherited disorder that affects about 1 in every 60,000 newborns. Babies suffering from galactosaemia are unable to process galactose, one of the simple sugars formed by the digestion of the milk sugar lactose. There may be no indication of a problem when the baby first nurses, as galactosaemia is only diagnosable through newborn screening. Eventually the galactose builds up to dangerous levels, where damage to the liver, central nervous system, eyes and kidneys can occur. Babies with galactosaemia should never be fed breastmilk or ordinary infant formulas. Your paediatrician will recommend a special diet.

Because galactosaemia is a recessive genetic trait, both parents can carry the gene without any symptoms. If anyone in your family has a history of galactosaemia, tell your doctor immediately. Your doctor might recommend genetic counselling before pregnancy or delivery. Newborns can be checked for galactosaemia as a matter of routine with a simple blood test. Make sure your child is tested.

Kari gave birth to her long-awaited daughter just before the New Year, but Lauren was born with meconium stain and was suctioned with a tube to clear her throat. She was slow to nurse, but suctioning, coupled with newborn jaundice, was thought to be the cause. They came home on New Year's Eve.

What is a meconium stain?
Meconium is your baby's first stool. It consists of swallowed amniotic fluid and excess cellular matter. Usually babies pass meconium after birth. However, sometimes meconium is passed in utero and can be inhaled by the baby, causing respiratory distress.

Because Lauren had lost 10 per cent of her birth weight, Kari was determined to nurse. With the assistance of a lactation consultant and the support of a wonderful paediatrician, Kari expressed her milk and finger-fed her baby. Lauren began to gain weight, but just as she was learning to feed at the breast, Kari received an urgent call from her doctor.

Eight days after birth, Lauren was identified through newborn screening to be presumptively positive for galactosaemia. Usually the test would have been back within two days, but because of the New Year holiday weekend, it took six.

Until further testing could be completed, Lauren was put on a soya formula. For several weeks Kari expressed and froze her milk in the event that breastfeeding could continue. However, further testing confirmed that Lauren was galactosaemic.

Kari has become an advocate for families affected by galactosaemia. Lauren continues to thrive under her parents' informed and loving care.

PKU

Phenylketonuria (PKU) is a genetic condition found in 1 in every 16,000 newborns. Babies with PKU are unable to produce an enzyme that allows their bodies to absorb the amino acid phenylalanine. Dangerous levels of phenylalanine can build up in a PKU baby's body, causing symptoms ranging from rashes to central nervous system damage.

Babies with PKU require frequent monitoring of their amino acid levels. They need just enough phenylalanine for growth, but an excess can be toxic. Breastmilk contains lower levels of phenylalanine than regular formula but is still not safe for exclusive feeding of a PKU baby. However, a combination of breastfeeding and a special infant formula is possible for these infants. Under supervision, you may be able to breastfeed a little bit every day.

If you have PKU and are pregnant, you need to pay close attention to your diet. Even if your baby doesn't inherit the condition, high levels of phenylalanine in your blood can cause serious harm to your unborn child.

CHAPTER 3

Breasts and Milk Production

You have the incredible ability to nourish your child exclusively from your own body for the first six months of his or her life. Lactation is an amazing gift that benefits both you and your baby in many ways. Although you don't necessarily need to know how the process works to be a successful breast-feeding mother, you might be surprised at just how miraculous the process of lactation is.

Breast Development

Breast buds begin developing in female embryos just four weeks after conception. By the time of birth, basic breast development is complete. The nipples, areolae and even some milk ducts are in place, along with a small pad of fat. Everything is functional on a very small scale.

From just after birth until puberty, breast development is almost on hold. Some milk ducts and glandular tissue grow, but the process doesn't really take off until 10–14 years of age.

Some babies leak breastmilk at birth. In the past, people called this 'witches' milk'. Far from being some kind of unnatural event, however, such leakage is normal and not uncommon. The pregnancy hormones in your body that prepare you for lactation can also cause your newborn's breasts to produce milk. The hormones typically leave the baby's body in a few days and the symptoms pass.

At the onset of puberty, a hormone called oestrogen is secreted by the ovaries, bringing about a rush of breast development. The mammary fat pad increases in size, and the milk ducts grow longer and branch out. When the menstrual cycle begins, the hormone progesterone causes the development of breast alveoli, the milk-producing cells.

By the age of 20, the process is nearly complete. However, breasts actually continue to mature until either pregnancy or the age of 30–35. Some women may wonder why, with all this growth, their breasts aren't larger. The important thing to remember is that breast development is your body's way of preparing you to nourish a baby. The size of your breasts does not affect your ability to produce milk – breast size is actually determined by heredity and body fat, and has very little to do with your ability to nurse.

Childbirth naturally completes the cycle of breast development.

Breast Anatomy

A basic knowledge of breast anatomy is helpful in understanding milk production. Think of your lactating breasts as a kind of fruit salad. This sounds weird, but it will make sense in a minute.

The insides of your breasts are divided into sections like the inside of a grapefruit. Each of these sections is called a lobe. Every breast has 15–25 lobes. Inside each lobe are 20–40 smaller sections called lobules. The lobules contain the glands that produce milk. Those glands are called alveoli and they cluster together like grapes around the milk ducts. The milk ducts join together like grape stems and connect to the milk sinuses located under the areola.

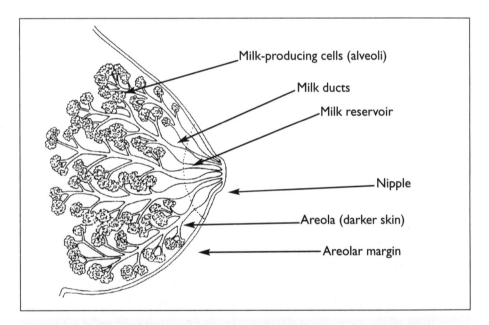

FIGURE 3-1: Internal organization. The clusters of alveoli produce milk and the ducts transport it to the sinuses, where your breastmilk is stored until your baby's next feeding.

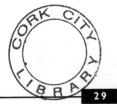

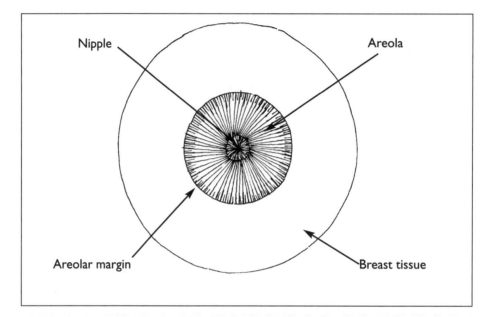

FIGURE 3-2: External diagram. The breast is divided into three sections. The areola is vitally important for successful breastfeeding.

Your Changing Breasts

With the onset of your first pregnancy, your breasts get their marching orders. The placenta stimulates your body to produce hormones (oestrogen and progesterone) that prepare your breasts for lactation. Recent animal research indicates that the placenta itself may actually produce those hormones. Your body responds to this call in several ways.

First, your nipples and areolae darken. This helps them to stand out from the surrounding tissue and act as a visual bull's-eye for your baby. Dramatic experiments in Europe highlighted the importance of the areola's darkening. After delivery, babies were placed face-down on their mother's abdomen. Amazingly, those little newborns zoomed in on their mother's nipples, crawled up and latched onto a breast without any direction or assistance – all from an infant who wouldn't know how to control her own body for months yet. This incredible inborn ability disappears soon after a baby's first hour of life.

Second, your breasts grow larger and sometimes tender. Throughout pregnancy, some women gain well over 680g (1½lb) in each breast as glandular tissue is being added to enable lactation. These milk-producing cells will replace a large portion of the fat cells in your breasts.

Third, your milk ducts grow. These ducts are the paths milk takes from the dairy in the alveoli to the sinuses under your areolae. Your breasts are doing road construction during pregnancy, increasing both the number of ducts and their size.

Finally, your Montgomery glands become noticeable as bumps on your areolae. These glands produce an oily substance that cleans and lubricates your nipples.

Studies indicate that women who have been pregnant enjoy a decreased risk of breast cancer compared to women who have never been pregnant. These findings imply that your breasts are just like the rest of your body in one important way – they are healthier when used the way nature intended.

At some point in your second trimester, the work is done and your breasts are ready to nourish your baby. The high levels of progesterone in your body prevent lactation from occurring before birth, but you may notice a fluid leaking from your breasts. This fluid is called colostrum, and it varies from thin and clear to thick and white. Colostrum is formed when the cells inside your new milk glands dissolve. Some women leak a little colostrum during pregnancy and others don't – either situation is perfectly normal.

How Your Breasts Produce Milk

Breasts are not like bottles; they aren't just containers for milk. Your breasts are never empty, and you don't need to wait until you feel full to nurse. Milk is manufactured constantly, as long as there is demand. Milk production, or lactogenesis, normally begins with the birth of your baby. Labour and delivery start a physiological chain reaction. The expulsion of your placenta causes the levels of the hormones oestrogen and progesterone in your body to fall. At the same time, nerve impulses from the uterus travel to the brain's hypothalamus gland. The brain then signals the pituitary gland to release the hormones prolactin and oxytocin.

Extra blood is sent to your breasts so they can start manufacturing milk. It's this extra blood, along with your milk coming in, that starts to engorge your breasts, sometimes painfully.

The prolactin released by your pituitary gland causes the grapelike clusters of alveoli to produce milk. The other hormone, oxytocin, aids in the ejection of milk from the breast.

It usually takes about 72 hours for your breasts to begin producing abundant milk. The process is completely under way within five days. During the first day or two of his life, your baby is nourished not with milk, but with your colostrum, the ideal first food for your infant.

Although your milk will come in after birth whether your child nurses or not, only the constant removal of milk from the breast can maintain milk production once you begin to lactate. Your baby's suckling signals your pituitary gland to release more oxytocin and prolactin. Just as in the beginning, these hormones cause your breasts to produce milk. If your baby drinks less milk than your breast produces, the excess milk remaining in your breasts will reduce future milk production.

It's a wonderfully self-regulating system: the more your child nurses, the more milk you produce; the less your child nurses, the less milk you produce. So, if you're worried about your milk supply, the solution is simply to nurse more often. Allowing your baby to nurse whenever she wants is also the best way to increase your milk supply.

Supplementing breastmilk with formula short-circuits the whole process. Anything that reduces your baby's hunger or her need to suck will ultimately reduce your milk supply. That's why glucose, water, formula and even dummies are not recommended for breastfeeding babies – your baby needs to be hungry and eager to suckle when you put her to breast.

Breastmilk Contents

You might wonder what's so special about breastmilk. Actually, there are hundreds of ingredients identified in breastmilk that are missing from infant formula, while other ingredients are found in different concentrations. Human milk is unique and cannot be duplicated; its ingredients have been tailored by millions of years of evolution to help human babies survive. However, even if every ingredient in human milk could be duplicated, breastmilk would still have significant advantages over formula.

Remarkably, your milk is alive. It's almost more like white blood than milk. Like blood, your milk is rich in antibodies that fight infections in your baby. Living cells from your body, called macrophages, enter your child's body through breastfeeding. These macrophages cruise through your baby's system gobbling up germs, which is especially important during the first months of life, when your baby's own immune system is weak.

Your own milk also contains living enzymes that help your baby digest her meal. Formula can't do that. Neither can the cows' milk most formulas are based on. Of the hundreds of different kinds of animal milks, only human breastmilk is perfectly suited for human babies.

A PARTIAL COMPARISON OF HUMAN MILK AND COWS' MILK

Carbohydrates	lactose	breastmilk has almost twice as much as cows' milk
	oligosaccharides	12 times as much as cows' milk
Proteins	caseins	less than a tenth of the amount of cows' milk
	lactalbumin	twice as much as cows' milk
	lactoferrin	present in human milk, but only trace amounts in cows' milk
	secretory immunoglobulin A (IgA)	70 times as much as cows' milk
	lactoglobulin	none in human milk, but present in cows' milk; can lead to dietary protein allergy
Minerals	sodium, potassium and magnesium	a third the amount of cows' milk
	chloride	half as much as cows' milk
	calcium	a quarter the amount of cows' milk

Human breastmilk is rich in the carbohydrates needed to fuel your child's active body and brain. Up to 40 per cent of the calories in human milk comes from the milk sugar lactose. Human milk gets more of its energy content from lactose than any other animal milk. Lactose gives your milk a sweet taste and won't cause diarrhoea, as the processed sugars in formula might.

Baby-Friendly Food

The proteins in human milk are also friendlier to your baby's digestive system. Most of the protein in cows' milk is in the form of casein, which forms hard curds in your baby's stomach. Breastmilk proteins are more easily absorbed and put less of a strain on your baby's system. One protein, immunoglobulin A, seals your baby's intestinal tract against allergens and infections. Another, lactoferrin, keeps iron away from the germs in your baby's body so they can't use it to reproduce.

The protein in our food is broken down by digestion into compounds called amino acids. Amino acids are the building blocks used to construct and maintain your body. Breastmilk contains ideal levels of taurine, an amino acid that builds and maintains the brain and eyes. Human milk also contains just the right levels of phenylalanine and tyrosine, while cows' milk and formula have too much. Excessive amounts of these two amino acids can lead to a serious medical condition in infants called PKU (see Chapter 2).

fact

Amino acids build cells, form antibodies, carry oxygen, aid in cell reproduction and muscle operation, and perform many other tasks in the human body. There are 22 known amino acids. Eight cannot be manufactured in the body, and these are called the essential amino acids and must come from dietary sources. Milk, cheese, eggs and meat are good sources of the essential amino acids for a breastfeeding mother.

Another vital ingredient in infant nutrition is fat. Fats and cholesterol are especially important to your baby's brain and nervous system development, and your breastmilk has all he needs. Human milk is your baby's only source for the important brain-builder docosahexaenoic acid (DHA). Breastmilk is also low in saturated fats and high in polyunsaturated fats: polyunsaturated fats help build brain and nerve cells, and saturated fats only help body growth. Research suggests that adequate levels of the right dietary fats might even help reduce your child's risk of developing diseases such as multiple sclerosis.

The balance of nutrients is also important. The mix of minerals and vitamins in human milk is carefully proportioned for human babies. An excess of any one vitamin or mineral can affect the body's absorption of other nutrients or encourage harmful bacteria to grow. Breastmilk provides nutrients in both a form and an amount that your child's body can easily use.

Nature designed the breastfeeding mechanisms so well that they respond to your baby's changing dietary needs. At different times in your baby's life, and even at different moments during a feeding, the composition of your milk changes.

Colostrum

Colostrum is the first milk your breasts produce. It's powerful stuff that is just what your newborn needs. Colostrum contains more protein, minerals, salt, vitamin A, nitrogen, white blood cells and antibodies than mature milk. It's also lower in fat and sugar. Frequent feedings of colostrum help your baby get off to a great start. You'll produce about two tablespoons of colostrum in the first 24 hours after birth – just the right amount for your baby's tiny tummy. In addition to the nutritional benefits, colostrum also helps clean the meconium from your newborn's intestines. Meconium causes your baby's stools to have the appearance and consistency of tar – this is a natural occurrence, but one that we're all happy to see end. The speedy elimination of meconium reduces the risk of jaundice in your newborn.

Preterm Milk

Preterm milk is produced if you give birth to a premature child. This milk is high in fats, proteins and sugars to help your baby grow and gain weight. After about a month, preterm milk changes into mature milk. Your body's ability to formulate the right quality of milk for your baby is nothing short of amazing.

Transitional Milk

Transitional milk is the mixture of colostrum and mature milk that your breasts produce between birth and the time your mature milk comes in. Transitional milk still has an extra advantage to it because of its colostrum content. As time passes, it gives way to your mature milk.

Mature Milk

Mature milk begins to come in within 72 hours of birth and normally replaces transitional milk completely within five days postpartum. Your mature breastmilk will exclusively provide your baby with all of her nutritional needs for the first six months of life. Mature breastmilk is actually more than a single substance – your baby receives two types of milk at each feeding: foremilk and hindmilk.

Foremilk

Foremilk is the milk that collects in the breast between feedings. About one-third of the milk your baby drinks at each feeding will be foremilk; it's the first course of your baby's meal. Foremilk satisfies her need for water and energy. It's like a quick pick-me-up, but it doesn't contain everything a growing baby needs. For a complete feeding, your baby needs to nurse long enough on one breast to get the hindmilk.

Hindmilk

Hindmilk is the main course. It's rich in nutrients and fats, both of which your baby needs to grow. Almost two-thirds of the human brain is composed of fat; brain and nervous system development depends on fat, and your hindmilk delivers it. The richness of hindmilk also gives your baby a satisfied, full feeling that helps her know she's had enough to eat.

Foremilk and hindmilk work together to customize the breastfeeding experience throughout your lactation. When your baby isn't really hungry but wants to nurse for emotional closeness, she receives only low-fat foremilk, and the same is true for older babies who nurse less frequently.

Milk Ejection Reflex or Letdown

The release of milk caused by oxytocin is called the letdown reflex or the milk ejection reflex. When your baby suckles, the stimulation to the nipple signals your body to release oxytocin, the hormone responsible for milk ejection. The oxytocin reaches your breast tissue, where it causes the tiny muscles surrounding the milk-producing glands to contract. The milk is forced down the milk ducts to the sinuses beneath your areolae. When your baby nurses, she compresses the milk sinuses and the milk is pushed through the holes in your nipple.

It takes a few moments after the start of nursing for letdown to occur. Fifty per cent of women will know the moment it happens, and the other 50 per cent won't. You might feel a tingling in your breasts, or even a pins and needles sensation. This feeling is followed by a sudden release of milk. Some women will experience multiple milk ejection reflexes during a single feeding. Sometimes letdown occurs when you are away from your baby, and when this happens, milk can shoot out in streams. Major tip: nursing pads – don't leave home without them!

Oxytocin production can be easily influenced by your state of mind – if you're stressed or distracted, your letdown reflex might be delayed or inhibited. Other factors that might affect letdown include cold, pain, fatigue, caffeine and nicotine. Fortunately, the prolactin you produce when the baby suckles is a natural tranquillizer.

Once you have letdown, you'll feel thirsty, relaxed and drowsy. You'll also feel your uterus contract. This is sometimes referred to as 'afterpains', and the contractions will decrease in intensity with time.

With letdown, you might notice your milk flowing faster and your baby swallowing more frequently. Even if you can't feel it, if you can see and hear your baby swallow, you'll know it's happened.

Often in the morning, when milk is most abundant, your infant may gag or cough. You can decrease the flow of milk by altering positions.

Breast and Nipple Care

Your breast is almost like a self-cleaning oven. The Montgomery glands surrounding your nipples secrete an oily substance that keeps your breasts clean and moist. There is very little you need to do. In fact, overzealous cleansing of your nipples can lead to problems, where soap will dry your nipple and can cause painful cracking. Soap also leaves unpleasant-tasting residue on your skin.

When bathing, use plain water to wash your breasts and nipples. If you wash your hands before and after each feeding, your breasts will stay clean. After nursing, rub some breastmilk over your areola. Your milk has medicinal properties that will help keep your nipple healthy. Then, if possible, let your nipples air dry.

Use plain water when washing your breasts. Avoid soaps and gels, even in the shower. Your nipples produce natural oils that cleanse and moisturize the areola; soap will remove these oils and can cause problems for nursing.

If you wear nursing pads, change them often, as warm, dark and wet pads are an ideal breeding ground for germs. The best pads are washable, breathable cotton; nursing pads with waterproof liners only hold the moisture in.

CHAPTER 4

Prenatal Preparation

Forewarned is forearmed (and you'll wish you had four arms!). Try to take advantage of the free time that you enjoy now to get prepared for feeding your newborn. Fortunately, there are lots of things you can do now to make breastfeeding more successful and less stressful. Now is the time to get yourself up to that starting line and get set to go – you'll be glad that you did.

Nipple Assessment

One of the first steps towards breastfeeding success is determining your nipple type. You can do this by conducting a nipple self-assessment. Roll your nipple between your fingers, have your partner stimulate your breasts, or open the freezer and stand in the cold air. How do your nipples react? Each single nipple is different, even when it's on the same person. Regardless of your nipple type, you can still breastfeed.

Inverted Nipples

Nipples become inverted due to tight connective tissue bands under the areola. Inverted nipples appear to dent inwards. (Flat nipples are caused by the same restrictive bands.) Both of these nipple types make it difficult for babies to latch on. It's still possible to breastfeed, but this might take a little extra effort. You can safely evert your nipples under the guidance of your lactation consultant. One of two methods will usually draw them out.

FIGURE 4-1:
Breast shell

FIGURE 4-2:
Hoffman's
Technique

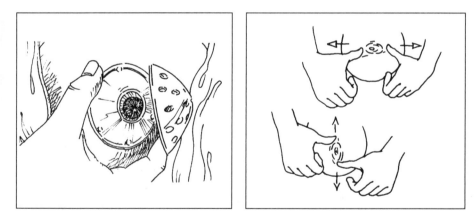

Breast shells – Breast shells are a wonderful invention for mothers who want to nurse but have inverted or flat nipples. They look like little dome-shaped cups with holes in the middle. Breast shells are worn inside your bra and fit over the nipple to put gentle pressure on the breast's connective bands and push the nipple out and through the opening. Other holes provide ventilation to keep your nipples dry.

You can wear shells during the last trimester of your pregnancy for a couple of hours per day, gradually increasing to approximately 10 hours at a time. Once your baby is born, you can continue to use them. Breast shells don't hurt, and no one can tell you're wearing them. They also come in handy if you have sore nipples.

Hoffman's Technique – Another method used by midwives and lactation consultants is called Hoffman's Technique. Hoffman's helps to stretch the base of the nipple and gives your baby a more pliable area to latch onto. To practise this technique, place your thumbs on each side of your nipple; while gently pressing inwards, pull your thumbs away from each other in a stroking motion. Now position your thumbs near the top and bottom of your nipple and repeat. You can do this several times each day during the last trimester. Ask your doctor or midwife to demonstrate this exercise on your next visit.

Breast pumps – After your baby is born, you can use the suction of a breast pump to pull your nipple out just prior to putting baby to the breast, but only for as long as it takes to get the nipple erect. You need to use the pump only on the side the baby has difficulty latching onto. Remember, he is feeding from the breast, not the nipple, but he must be able to extend the nipple to the back of his throat. Any breastmilk expressed by the pump can be saved for later use.

Some women with flat or inverted nipples are able to feed without any nipple preparation at all. Often your baby will provide the best suction and the problem will take care of itself.

Nipple Preparation

It was once believed that nipples had to be 'toughened' to prepare for nursing. This is no longer considered to be best practice. Research has found that the cause of sore nipples isn't nursing friction, it's poor latch – in other words, the problem is how your baby takes the nipple into his mouth. When your baby latches onto your breast correctly, your nipples won't hurt.

The only thing you really need to do to prepare yourself for breastfeeding is to become familiar with your breasts. You might not be comfortable with this at first. Women are taught to be self-conscious about their bodies from childhood, and often feel embarrassed about the size and shape of their breasts. Not only do they wear bras to support the weight of their breasts, they sometimes wear them just to keep their breasts covered.

Don't overstimulate your nipples during these self-assessment techniques! Nipple stimulation during pregnancy can cause uterine contractions and, potentially, premature labour. STOP if you feel any contractions. If contractions do not subside, contact your health-care provider.

Our society has been so successful in sexualizing breasts that we have come to believe that they are purely sexual organs. Getting to know your breasts is education, not masturbation. This kind of self-exam is not unlike what women do to screen for breast cancer. All you have to do is give your breasts a mere fraction of the attention that your partner gives them, and you'll learn everything you need to know. Then you'll feel comfortable and be confident that these self-regulating wonders will provide ample nourishment for your baby.

Social–Emotional Preparation

Getting physically ready for your newborn is only the beginning. It's equally important to prepare yourself emotionally for this event that will change your life forever. Once your baby arrives, life as you know it is over. For the next year or more, you will truly understand the term 'joined at the hip', and in time, you'll wonder what life was like BC (Before Children). You will fall in love all over again and want to provide the very best that life has to offer for your new baby.

You've also made the commitment to breastfeed. What will this mean for you? Will you return to work in six weeks? Will you stay at home and exclusively nurse your baby? Now is the time to think about how breastfeeding will have an impact on these decisions and on your life.

If you're going back to work, think about where you will be able to express your milk. Talk to your employer about policies that support breastfeeding mothers. Seek out childcare providers who are breastfeeding-friendly and who will allow you to stop by for an afternoon feeding or at the very least provide your baby with your expressed milk. Talk to other nursing mothers about techniques they've used and ask them to share their stories – both good and hair-raising – with you. Get in touch with a lactation consultant and schedule an appointment before your baby arrives. Search the Web for breastfeeding sites that offer the latest research. Find out what classes are offered within your community or join a breastfeeding mothers' group such as the La Leche League.

Begin to think of yourself as a breastfeeding parent!

Breastfeeding Supplies

At some point during your last trimester, your friends and family may ask what supplies and equipment would be useful during the first few months of the baby's life. Even if they don't, you'll need to go shopping for baby essentials. Don't forget the following.

Bras

When you head to the shopping centre or high street to buy a couple of comfortable nursing bras, you'll sigh as you pass Knickerbox or La Senza, wondering why they haven't picked up on this marketing opportunity. Then you'll head straight to the granny bra section of the nearest department store.

There are several styles of nursing bras to choose from, but your goal is to find a comfortable bra that supports your enlarged breasts and is easy to operate. Overleaf are a few factors to take into consideration.

FIGURE 4-3:
Nursing bra

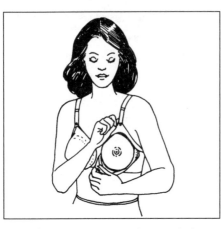

· Your cup size and bra (band) size will increase during pregnancy and will change when you nurse. You can expect to increase at least one size in each of these areas over the next couple of weeks.

· You'll be using the one-handed draw method for the next several months, so you'll need a bra that opens from the top to release the flap. Your new bra should also have adjustable straps, be easily breast-accessible and refasten in a single smooth swoop. With time, you'll be able to manoeuvre your bra blindfolded, which is what you'll be doing when you nurse in public.

· Comfort and support are crucial. Your bra should support not only your breasts, but part of your underarm, as your breast tissue extends beyond the obvious. Snug sports bras and other fashionable yet tight push-ups will send a signal to the brain to slow milk production and can also cause plugged ducts and breast infections.

· Unless you have very large or heavy breasts, underwired bras are unnecessary and best avoided. They can restrict milk production and flow. If you must purchase one, select a bra that fits properly and allows for room behind and beyond the milk ducts that extend past your armpits.

· Choose a breathable cotton bra without moisture-resistant liners. Trapped moisture can breed yeast or bacterial growth. If you intend to use nursing pads, it isn't necessary to have them built into your bra.

· Purchase a bra with several rows of hooks, or buy a bra extension to wear during the first two weeks – these are straps of fabric that are lined with additional hooks that fasten to the back of your bra and can turn a 36 band-size bra into a 40. Your breasts will change again once your routine is established, but for now you'll need a tool to support your expanding bustline.

When you find a bra that meets all of your criteria, buy two or three of the same kind. You'll be washing them frequently, so you'll want one available at any given time.

Pads

Nursing pads are a godsend for mothers with a fast milk ejection reflex. You may be standing in line at the supermarket when something triggers your letdown – maybe it's the sound or smell of an infant; maybe it's a picture of a baby – and your breasts achieve letdown like water pistols. Nursing pads are your protective barrier against public embarrassment. The most cost-effective pads are made of cotton or terry cloth and can be laundered and reused. Some are form-fitting to give you extra shapeliness.

All department stores sell nursing pads. They also market disposable pads with moisture-resistant plastic liners. When moisture gets trapped in the liners, bacteria and fungi can flourish in the warm, damp darkness. Who wants a petri dish in her bra? If you're on a budget, you can use cotton hankies or cut a cloth nappy to fit. Nursing pads just might give 'stuffing your bra' a whole new meaning.

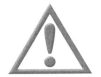

Cutting a disposable nappy into sections to use as nursing pads will release moisture beads that expand with wetness. These are difficult to remove from your breast and are easily ingested by your baby. Although the beads are not poisonous, they aren't meant for human consumption!

Pillows

You will use nursing pillows to help elevate your baby to your breast, and you'll also use them to support your arms and back. Most nursing pillows continue to be useful as your baby grows. At about five to six months, your baby can use your pillow for supported sitting.

Slings or Blankets

Slings are brilliant for discreet nursing in public, and they offer a convenient way to carry baby around the house. Most slings are made of a metre-long piece of cotton fabric that you can adjust to 'wear' your baby in several positions as he grows. (Most will hold up to about 17.5kg/35lb.) Traditionally, slings are used in countries where women continue to work with their baby attached at the hip. In the Western world, slings are a relatively new idea, but they've become the fashion choice for a wide variety of breastfeeders.

FIGURE 4-4:
Sling

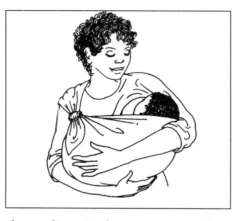

As with baby hammocks, slings support your baby's spine and keep it aligned. Research has shown that babies carried by sling, kept close to their parents, cry less, are more calm, have stronger attachment formation and are more in sync with their mother's movements.

You can wear double slings if you have twins. Think of them as baby bandoliers. The best part about slings is that you can walk around nursing your baby, and no one will know. You can opt to use blankets instead, and these are just as handy. They can easily be used to shelter a nursing baby and double as warmers in a cold car seat.

Pumps

If you plan to return to work, or just want a reliable breast pump, make your purchase now. There are many different types and brands, and you need to choose a model that's both efficient and cost-effective. Hiring is another option. Call your health visitor or an organization such as the NCT for information. The best breast pumps are quite expensive, but they are a good investment if you intend to use them regularly. Some women have purchased cheap, battery-operated handheld pumps that are simply not powerful enough for the task, while others have invested in professional- or hospital-grade pumps that grew cobwebs in the cupboard. Again, have a good idea of what your needs are, and choose the best pump for your circumstances.

Footstool

Babies need a lap to nurse. Create a comfortable lap by using a footstool, which eliminates stress on your legs, back and shoulders. You can improvise by using any item that's sturdy enough to support your feet and legs – try a coffee table, a pile of books or a cardboard box. If you're discussing the purchase of a new chair or sofa, a matching footstool is worth the extra money.

Breast Shells

Breast shells won't be necessary for everyone, but if you have flat or inverted nipples, they are an important purchase. They also help if you have sore or cracked nipples from improper latch. You can find these via specialist baby and mother shops or department stores, or you can buy them at most online baby equipment suppliers.

Burping Cloths

It's a time-honoured truth: babies are moist. Whether you breastfeed or bottle feed, your baby will spit up. A couple of dozen cloth nappies are a wise, inexpensive and necessary investment. Cloth nappies are thick, absorbent, and cost less than a new wardrobe.

Nursing Fashions

Once your baby arrives, you'll move into the exciting world of nursing fashions! You'll want to purchase two-piece outfits that allow for easy breast access. You can choose blouses that button or those that can be lifted. Oversized tops, sweatshirts, leggings, pedal pushers and Lycra become the nursing mother's uniform. Comfort is vital. You'll want to avoid dry clean-only fabrics and replace them with washable, breathable cottons and other fabrics that don't trap moisture. Prints tend to hide the telltale bull's-eyes of breastmilk leakage that solids only emphasize.

Labour Medications and Breastfeeding

Discuss labour pain management with your midwife or doctor, and ask your doctor what she recommends. During labour, you need to be free to concentrate on the task at hand and not on making last-minute decisions.

Your choices for pain relief will be either pharmacological (drugs) or non-pharmacological. Ask your provider to explain the risks and the benefits of the various methods she employs as well as the effects they have on breastfeeding – a fast, relatively easy labour might require only support and encouragement, while a long, difficult labour might require the use of many different options.

The most common types of pharmacological interventions include:

Gas and air. This combination of nitrous oxide gas and oxygen is inhaled via a mask, and you can administer the dose yourself as and when you feel you need it. The gas numbs the pain centre in the brain, and once the contraction has passed or you feel you can cope, you simply put the mask aside. This method can give you the sensation of floating, and some women have reported feeling nauseous. This is only a mild form of pain relief, but the effects are almost instant, and it won't affect the baby.

Pethidine. This morphine-based drug is administered via an injection into the thigh or buttock, and inhibits the brain's ability to register pain. These sorts of narcotics take about 20 minutes to work. Because pethidine crosses the placenta, it can can make your baby sleepy and slow to breathe, and as a result is not suitable for use too close to the actual birth. Once you have been given pethidine you will have to lie down, so active labour becomes impossible until the effects have worn off; it may also make you nauseous. However, pethidine can be valuable if you have a very long, drawn-out labour.

Epidural anaesthesia. Epidural anaesthesia consists of injections of small amounts of anaesthetics near the spinal nerves. This method eliminates pain in some areas of your body but allows you to remain alert throughout the birth of your baby. Unfortunately, it also weakens your contractions and slows labour. You often don't feel the urge to push, and the experience of giving birth is something you might feel you have missed.

Labour medications will cross the placental wall and enter your baby's bloodstream. The effects of these medications can cause your infant to have a delayed latch or uncoordinated suckling. Your baby may have a hard time getting to the breast if he's sleepy from drugs. Combining medications seems to increase this effect, especially for the first 12 hours after delivery.

The most common types of non-pharmacological interventions are:

Pattern-paced breathing. This type of breathing is a relaxation technique taught in childbirth class. Your mantra may start out as 'Hee hee hee ho' and end with 'I want to go home NOW!'

Hot-and-cold therapy. Heated rice socks, blankets and ice packs are natural ways of stopping pain receptors from signalling to the brain. They also provide competing sensations that decrease your awareness of pain.

Massage and acupressure. These techniques work in much the same way as hot-and-cold therapy. Acupressure stimulates a set of nerve impulses that interrupts pain signals. Massage relaxes and releases tension. Scented massage oils provide aromatherapy for the body and brain.

Changing positions. When you're on medication, you become a health risk and a hospital liability. That's why women in labour were traditionally confined to their hospital bed. Lying flat on your back throughout labour was not nature's plan. When you can walk or use a birthing ball, gravity assists you by expanding your pelvic cavity so your baby can descend more quickly and efficiently. Unrestricted movement decreases labour duration.

Water therapy. Hydrotherapy is a tool that relieves discomfort in labour. Water is relaxing in almost any form. It has proven effective in relieving high blood pressure and backache. Many women go into labour in the bath and give birth in special pools.

TENS machine. Transcutaneous Electrical Nerve Stimulation (TENS) is an increasingly popular form of pain relief. The small battery-operated machine is attached to your body with adhesive pads, rather like a body-toning device. A small electrical current is passed through your skin, reducing the pain messages being sent to your brain and stimulating feel-good endorphins. This is a non-invasive form of pain relief that can be used with any other method except in water, and you are free to move about while using it. You also have the advantage that you are in charge of the dial. Some hospitals have TENS machines, but many women opt to be sure by hiring one.

A large part of the decision you make about pain relief depends on your perspective and attitude about the birth process (is it a natural event or a medically managed condition?) and your confidence in your ability to be in labour and to give birth. Recently, a group of midwives found that fewer than half of the women who started labour naturally needed pain medication. Unmedicated births make for more alert babies who are eager to initiate breastfeeding and have a stronger, more coordinated suck.

Breastfeeding and Your Birth Plan

Hospitals are now striving to become more maternal-friendly. They encourage patients to be partners in their own health care. One way to accomplish this goal is through the use of birth plans.

Birth plans are written statements that allow you to make informed decisions about labour, delivery and newborn procedures before your baby arrives. They are based on both current information and available options. These plans open the door for communication with your doctor. There are interactive birth plans available on several websites.

It is important to remember that most plans are based on idealized births. Your birthing experience will almost certainly fall somewhere in the middle. You can plan for the best, but expect that there may be a revision or two, if medically necessary, and be flexible enough to allow for it.

The Nouns: People, Places and Things

When formulating your birth plan, you'll have several factors to consider, from who will be attending the birth, to where you hope to have it, to what labour methods you will use. Discuss your options with your partner and your doctor to determine what works best for you.

THE PEOPLE

Who will attend your birth?

Are partners, siblings and extended family welcome?

Will you use a doula (see page 53)?

Will staff and students be allowed to breeze in and out during the process?

Will your birth partner be present for all newborn care procedures?

THE PLACES

Will your labour take place at the hospital or at home?

Will you go into labour, give birth and recover in the same room?

Does this room come equipped with a squat bar, birthing bed or birthing pool?

Will the baby room with you fully, partially or not at all?

THE THINGS

Will you birth naturally or use medications?

What interventions are acceptable to you (induction, forceps, vacuum, internal foetal monitoring)?

What birth methods are approved and supported by your provider (birthing ball, full or restricted movement, hydrotherapy)?

Remember that a birthing plan is the starting point for you and your doctor. You'll be otherwise occupied during delivery, so it's important that the other people involved know your wishes and intentions.

Your Breastfeeding Plan

You will want to make a special note in your birth plan that you intend to breastfeed. It is important to have this in writing, but tell your doctor as well as the nursery staff. If you're using a doula, she will be the first to help your baby to the breast, and she will keep hospital staff informed.

You will want to include the following in your plan:

1. Please do not offer my baby formula, glucose (sugar water), dummies or artificial nipples.
2. My primary feeding preference is exclusive breastfeeding.
3. I would like assistance to help me establish a nursing routine before I leave the birthing facility.
4. In the event that my baby needs medical interventions, I would like to provide expressed breastmilk.

Some newborn-care nurses may recommend offering your baby a glucose or formula supplement. Get your partner to speak up for you.

Fathers are your greatest support! Your partner can make sure your baby isn't given dummies, formula or glucose, and he can stand up against hospital policies that aren't breastfeeding-friendly.

Sugar water and formula will fill your baby's stomach so he won't be hungry when you offer your breast for feeding. Babies given supplements aren't learning how to breastfeed – they are learning how to feed from a bottle. However, there are situations that might require supplementation with formula for medical emergencies (see Chapter 10). If your baby is unable to nurse, your doctor and midwife will work with you to express colostrum for use.

The use of dummies should also be identified in your birth plan. Dummies will satisfy your baby's sucking reflex, but you need your baby's suckle to help develop your milk supply, and dummies will only hinder this process. Dummies should not be introduced until at least six weeks after birth or until a solid nursing routine has been established.

The Use of Doulas

Many couples are now employing the services of qualified doulas to assist them with labour, birth and postnatal care. A prenatal doula is a professional labour assistant who:

- Acts as a liaison between medical staff and the labouring couple.
- Views childbirth as a natural event and not a medically managed condition.
- Guides your birth partner in providing natural relief, support and encouragement to you during labour.
- Helps you develop your birth plan and advocates for its use.
- Provides comfort measures.
- Records all aspects of your birth story.

Doulas are very much like nurturing Earth Mothers. Both mothers and fathers report more favourable birth experiences with the use of a qualified labour assistant. Dads often find the experience much more positive and pleasurable and far less stress -inducing when another person is present to share the task of providing comfort and support.

Both prenatal and postnatal doulas are available to help you establish a breastfeeding routine. Your prenatal doula won't leave your side until your baby is placed at your breast and latched on properly. Your postnatal doula will assist with newborn care, breastfeeding, emotional support and, sometimes, light household assistance. They provide home-based services because home is the environment where you will raise your baby.

Studies on the use of doulas have found a 50 per cent reduction in Caesarean rates, 25 per cent decrease in labour duration, 60 per cent reduction in epidural use, 40 per cent reduction in oxytocin induction, 30 per cent decrease in the need for medications, 40 per cent reduction in forceps deliveries, as well as fewer birth complications, lower rates of postnatal depression, increased breastfeeding success and greater reported satisfaction with the childbirth experience.

Most doulas charge around £250–500 for attending a birth, according to the experience of a doula. You can also hire a doula to help you post partum, and for this you can expect to pay £10–15 per hour. Doula UK is a network of doulas run voluntarily by doulas – *www.doula.org.uk* or write to Doula UK, PO Box 26678, London N14 4WB.

CHAPTER 5
Breastfeeding Basics

mmediately after birth and barring any complications, your doctor or midwife will lay your newborn on your abdomen, and you'll greet each other for the very first time. Your baby will be alert, and the sound of your voice will captivate her. She will turn her head to listen to her mother and father, and your voices will probably calm her cries within seconds. She might even try to respond to your soothing coos.

The First Hour

If breastfeeding is in your birth plan, your nurse or midwife will immediately place your baby at your breast to help involute your uterus and expel your placenta (or afterbirth). Nipple stimulation from your baby's suckling will cause your uterus to contract, which will gently squeeze the placenta to separate it from the uterine wall. It takes usually two to five contractions to deliver the placenta. Oxytocin is produced naturally when your baby nurses; it helps the uterus to contract, which controls blood loss and the risk of haemorrhage.

Newborns are superbly programmed for breastfeeding. They can zero in on the darkened bull's-eye of the areola and can see your face clearly while nursing at your breast. Babies nuzzle the nipple aggressively to make it erect for latching onto. They also have the ability to 'crawl' to the breast within the first hour after birth and to memorize the smell of your breastmilk.

While your care provider is busy delivering the placenta, clamping and cutting the umbilical cord, repairing any tears to the perineum and completing documentation, you and your baby will be exploring each other through rich sensory contact. You'll be counting her fingers and toes, and she'll be committing your scent to memory. Studies have shown that babies can identify their mothers from just the smell of their milk. Your baby is also satisfying her sucking reflex. This is the beginning of a beautiful relationship that will last a lifetime.

At the Hospital

In your birth plan, you noted that you intended to breastfeed. If you haven't already, now is the time to meet with a lactation consultant, someone who is a professional in the art of breastfeeding. Lactation consultants take international board exams to become licensed to practise, just as lawyers take the bar exam to practise law. They're recognized as top-level professionals in their field.

Hospitals will have experienced staff available to assist you, but in smaller or rural facilities, postnatal care nurses or certified breastfeeding educators will assist you if a lactation consultant is unavailable. These talented and caring people are there to instruct you in every aspect of breastfeeding, from positioning to latch to assessment. They'll show you how to nurse your baby and will provide support because they want you to succeed! If you or your partner happen to have a video camera handy, tape their demonstrations. They'll be invaluable when you go home and are on your own.

Ask

Ask questions. No question is too silly, stupid or small. If the answer is vague or you just don't understand, ask your lactation consultant to slow down and speak in real-world terms. Don't hesitate to seek clarification. Get your partner, a member of your family or another support person to take notes for you, or take this book with you and jot notes in the margins.

If you are unclear about anything, ask again. Don't be intimidated by a busy hospital or a buzzing nurse. This is your time – what you learn now can determine your immediate breastfeeding success.

Watch

Observe and pay close attention as your nurse demonstrates positions and steps involved in putting your baby to your breast. Remember throughout all this that reading about a technique and watching it in action are two completely different things.

Listen

The staff will share vital information with you. Stop what you're doing, make eye contact, and actively listen to what the person has to say. Draw pictures in your mind as she explains the process.

Practise

Practise, then practise again. We retain 90 per cent of what we're learning when we can demonstrate it and talk about it at the same time. Go through each step and describe what you are doing and why it is important to you.

Hospital staff will bring the baby to you for feeding every two to three hours around the clock. If your baby is staying in the room with you, the hospital staff will remind you to nurse often. This will increase your milk supply and will help you retain what you've learned about breastfeeding.

Before you leave the medical facility, inquire about hospital-grade breast pump hire. Ask the staff or a lactation consultant to recommend a model and to demonstrate its use. If you return to work and want to express your milk, or have a special needs baby and need to pump, you'll want a high-quality breast pump for home and/or business use. Pumps come in all makes and models (see Chapter 12.) Your lactation consultant can show you the best pumps to purchase or hire.

At Home

When you first arrive home with your new baby, you might feel a little nervous or awkward about breastfeeding on your own. 'Test anxiety' is perfectly normal when you're doing it for the first time on your own.

First and foremost, relax! Feel confident in your ability to do this! Keep this book close by for reference, and feel free to contact your postnatal nurse or lactation consultant for a final run-through. The first couple of weeks take practice, but by the time you go in for your postnatal check-up, you'll have nursing down to an art.

When to Feed

You'll receive a lot of advice (wanted or not) about how to feed your baby over the next couple of months. You'll be asked if you are feeding 'on schedule' or 'on demand': the latter is a term used to describe your baby's biological cycle; 'on schedule' usually means by the clock. In the first few days after birth, you will be doing both.

Frequency

How often you feed will be determined by your baby. If she is allowed to follow her own body rhythms throughout her life, she is less likely to be an overweight adult. Feeding on demand will also establish a strong milk supply. Babies know when they are hungry. They will demonstrate hunger cues when they are ready to eat. In simple terms, babies eat when they are hungry and they stop when they are full. The only clock your baby cares about is her own body clock.

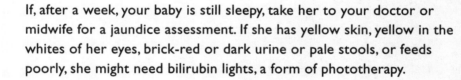

If, after a week, your baby is still sleepy, take her to your doctor or midwife for a jaundice assessment. If she has yellow skin, yellow in the whites of her eyes, brick-red or dark urine or pale stools, or feeds poorly, she might need bilirubin lights, a form of phototherapy.

At the same time, babies in their first week of life are very sleepy, particularly if labour medications were used during the birth process. If your baby isn't waking on her own every two to three hours during the first week, you'll need to wake her to breastfeed. Now you're feeding on schedule or by the clock.

After the first week of life, your baby will be more wakeful and will begin to tune into her own body rhythms. Until then, you will have to rouse her to reinforce the feeding pattern.

Schedule

During the early days, you'll realize that there is no schedule. Your baby has her own internal gauge. Her body will tell her when she's hungry, and she'll show you by demonstrating hunger cues. Your baby is ready to eat when she performs these actions:

·   Brings her clenched fist to her mouth
·   Begins sucking on her fist or fingers
·   Roots by turning her head to find your nipple
·   Displays increased activity or movement
·   Vocalizes and begins to make noise.

Crying is a late hunger cue. If you wait until babies cry, you've waited too long. Identifying early hunger cues is an important part of learning to 'read' your baby's behaviour. Knowledge is power. Anticipate that she will be hungry when she wakes up, or when she displays these cues.

How Long to Feed

Offer one breast first, and when baby is finished, offer the second. Women were once advised to let their babies nurse for just 10 minutes at each breast, but recent research suggests that the Ten Minute Rule no longer applies. The composition of breastmilk changes during a single feeding session and your baby needs both the foremilk and the hindmilk you produce. The foremilk comes quickly and is higher in volume and protein and lower in fat. The hindmilk is higher in fat and calories, but there's less of it. It's like having steak and ice cream, dinner and dessert. Babies need both.

Alternate the starting line-up at each feeding. Your baby might prefer one breast to the other, and that's normal. This might have to do with the position you hold her, the flow of milk or any number of factors. You might prefer one breast to the other for the same reasons. However, it is essential to alternate your breasts to ensure a good milk supply.

Feed for as long as your baby is interested; 15–30 minutes on average. If your baby is a marathon nurser on one breast, it could indicate that she is not latched on properly or there's a problem with your milk supply. However, babies approach nursing differently. It's a lot like eating ice-cream... some of us lick and savour it, while others bite and swallow. It rarely takes more than a maximum of 20 minutes per breast to 'empty' it. Some babies will continue to nurse for comfort.

> **tips**
>
> Most experts will tell you to feed your infant for 15 minutes on each breast, but you should watch your baby and not the clock. It's more important for your baby to remove your milk than it is to follow a predetermined time limit.

Breastmilk is very digestible, so breastfed babies eat more often than formula-fed babies. In the first weeks, your baby will eat smaller amounts, but frequently. Later on, your baby will eat more and will reduce the number of feedings. Growth spurts happen around three weeks, six weeks, three months and six months, and usually last about seven to ten days. During this time, you might notice that your baby eats more, and more frequently. Frequent feedings not only satisfy your baby, but they tell your body to make more milk in preparation for your baby's growing demands.

Baby at Your Breast: The Basics

Are you ready to begin? Eventually, both you and your baby will be old professionals. Until you've mastered your technique, however, follow these simple steps for successful breastfeeding. With practice and patience, you'll be nursing like a pro in no time!

Getting Ready

It's important to remember to wash your hands just before nursing. The Montgomery glands will keep your nipples clean, but it's essential to practise good hygiene when handling both your breasts and your newborn.

Don't forget your water! There's something about nursing that makes women thirsty, so have a beverage available. Water is the best choice, but juice or decaffeinated teas are healthy, too. Avoid caffeine, as it can reduce your milk supply and cause stomach upset for your baby.

Find a comfortable place that will become your nursing nest: a couch, a rocking chair or your bed. Use pillows to support your elbows, arms and back. Use a footrest, a telephone book or last week's washing to support your feet. Rocking chairs with footrests are perfect, but feel free to improvise with what you have available. It's important that you're comfortable. You may be there for a while.

Get Your Co-star

Bring your baby close to you, chest to breast, using the position that works best for both of you. Your baby's body will face you. Use pillows to bring her up to the level of your breast. Nursing pillows, bed pillows, rolled blankets, baby slings or sofa cushions will offer your baby support and the height she needs. It's important that when you are chest to breast with your baby, her ear, shoulder and hip form a straight line. Turn your head and try to swallow. It's not easy and it's uncomfortable! That's why it's important to have your baby's body aligned (ear, shoulder, hip).

Bring your baby to the breast, not the breast to your baby. Don't lean forwards to offer your breast. Instead, with one hand cradling her head, your forearm supporting her back and hips, and the other hand holding your breast, pull your baby to you.

Support your breast with a C hold, like the way you hold a hamburger, only upside down. When we eat, we use our hands to shape and contour the sandwich. The same principles apply here. Support your breast with your thumb on top positioned behind the areola and the weight of your breast in your hand. After a while, you might not need to continue this hold throughout the entire feeding, but if you have large or heavy breasts, they'll benefit from the support. If your hand seems awkward, place a rolled-up towel under your breast for support.

The All-Important Latch

Encourage her to open her mouth as wide as possible, as if she were yawning. You can tickle her cheek or bottom lip to stimulate her rooting reflex, if needed. In one sweeping motion, pull baby towards you to position her at your breast. Centre your nipple over your baby's tongue, aim your nipple towards the roof of her mouth and bring her chin to your breast.

Latching on correctly is the most critical key to breastfeeding success. This part takes some practice. Your baby should take the entire nipple and most of the areola into her mouth. If you have large areolae, make sure she's getting about 2.5cm (1in) of it into her mouth. More areola should be visible at the top of your breast than at the bottom. Latching on is not symmetrical. Note where her lower lip makes contact. It's the lower jaw that actually extracts the milk as she compresses the milk sinuses. Your nipple should be centred over her tongue. If it just doesn't feel right or it hurts, pull baby's lower lip back enough to see if her tongue is properly positioned over her lower gum line. If you can't see it, or if you hear a clicking noise when she nurses, she might be sucking her tongue in addition to your breast. Break the latch and reposition.

Your baby will take your nipple to the back of her throat. As she works her bottom jaw to compress the milk sinuses, milk trickles down the back of her throat. It's similar to the way you would suck your thumb.

FIGURE 5-1:
A proper latch

FIGURE 5-2:
Breaking
the latch

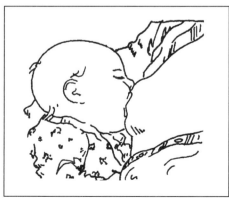
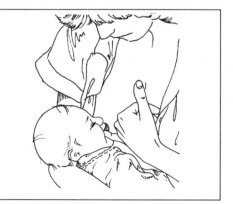

Breaking the Latch

Break the latch by inserting your finger into your baby's mouth at the inside cheek to release suction. Hook the nipple and draw it out as you pull your breast away. Baby might try to relatch, but if your hooked finger is covering your nipple, she can't. If you allow your baby to slide off the nipple while she's still creating suction, you'll have sore or cracked nipples. Breaking the latch will be a smooth process once you have tried it a couple of times.

LATCH EVALUATION CHECKLIST

❑ Does your baby have the entire nipple and at least 2.5cm (1in) of the areola in her mouth?

❑ After your milk lets down, can you hear your baby swallow?

❑ Does baby follow a 'suck, suck, suck, swallow' pattern?

❑ Do you hear a clicking sound that indicates improper latch?

❑ Can you see noticeable movement in her jaw all the way to her ear (ear wiggling)?

❑ Is the area at her temple moving?

❑ Are her lips flanged or everted around the nipple?

If you feel pain (excluding the tingling sensation of letdown), break the latch and reposition. If your baby is taking in only the nipple, break the latch and reposition. If something just doesn't feel right, break the latch and reposition.

Breastfeeding should not be painful. If your baby is positioned on your areola correctly, you should not feel anything more than a slight tug. Pain is often the result of nipple feeding, and continued nipple feeding will lead to cracked or sore nipples and even greater discomfort.

Suck, Suck, Suck, Swallow

Babies breastfeed in rhythm. At first they suck steadily and somewhat aggressively to stimulate your milk ejection reflex. As the jaw moves up and down against the breast sinuses to extract milk, you'll begin to notice a pattern to your baby's nursing. She might suck from four to 10 times, pause for about five or 10 seconds, then continue this pattern for about three to five minutes. This pattern stimulates the letdown of your hindmilk. Once this happens, you will be able to hear her swallow. Her rhythm changes to suck, suck, suck, swallow, pause, suck, suck, suck, swallow, pause. Once breastfeeding is established, letdown happens more quickly.

The flow of a fast milk ejection reflex can sometimes be more than your baby can handle. You might notice milk dripping from her mouth, or she might cough and need to catch her breath. If she's spluttering, break the latch and take her off the breast just long enough for her to swallow, then begin again. After a few minutes you'll notice that her suck will begin to slow and she'll have longer pauses between sucks.

As babies tire and begin to nod off, there will be several very long pauses. But the minute you try to take your baby off the breast or stimulate her cheek, she'll almost always start to suck again. Often, by this time, baby has slid off the areola and is nipple feeding, not breastfeeding. Break the latch and start again.

Labour Again?

Early on, you will feel uterine contractions when your baby begins to nurse. These are called afterpains. You might feel a gush of blood on your sanitary pad at the same time. With nipple stimulation, your uterus regains its tone and dispels excess blood. These same contractions also shrink your uterus to its pre-pregnant pear size.

If this is your second or third baby, your contractions might feel stronger than before. Practise the breathing patterns you used in childbirth education classes. After a few weeks, these contractions will cease.

Ending a Feeding

When your baby is done with the first breast, burp her, change her nappy if necessary, then offer her the second breast. However, she might fall asleep without finishing the second breast. It will be important to remember to start on the unfinished side the next time your baby nurses.

Breastfeeding Positions

After your baby arrives, both of you will find a technique that works for you. You'll also discover your preference for positions after some practice.

It is important that you feel comfortable with at least one of the positions listed below. Below are a few different options for you to try.

Cradle Position

The cradle position is the most commonly used position during the first few weeks of life. Because we tend to be cautious about holding our newborns, we tend to choose positions that allow us more control. In the cradle position, as in all breastfeeding positions, the baby's ear, shoulder and hip will form a line and baby will be chest to breast with you. Chest to breast means that you turn your baby towards you so her chest is even with your breast (and sometimes her foot will be in your armpit if she's especially active). Use pillows to cushion your baby in your lap. Baby needs to have her head and mouth at the same height as your nipple.

Your baby's head will be on your forearm (at the crook of your elbow), and her back will be along your inner arm. The palm of your hand will support her bottom. If you are preparing to breastfeed on the left breast, your right hand supports the breast in a C hold. You support your baby with your left arm and hand. Pull your baby to the breast with your forearm. Use pillows to cushion your elbows.

FIGURE 5-3:
Cradle hold

FIGURE 5-4:
Cross-cradle
position

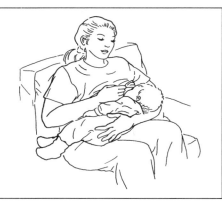
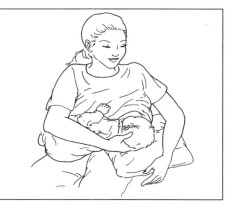

Cross-Cradle Position

This is another excellent method and the one used most frequently while learning the art of breastfeeding. The cross-cradle gives you maximum control in holding your baby and bringing her to the breast. If nursing on the right side, gently place your left hand behind your baby's ears with your thumb and index finger, behind each ear. Your baby's neck rests in the web between the thumb, index finger and palm of your hand. The palm of your hand is positioned between her shoulder blades. Your right hand supports your breast in the C position.

Again, use pillows to support baby and your arms. As you begin the latch, make sure baby's mouth is close to your nipple and at the same height. When baby opens her mouth, bring her to your nipple with the palm of your hand from between her shoulder blades.

Football Hold

This is a great position for a mother who has had a Caesarean birth, has large breasts, or has a very large or premature baby. Most newborns are comfortable in this position, too. To use the football hold, place baby on her side at your side. You support your baby's head in your hand and her back along your arm as you did in the cross-cradle hold, but this time the baby is beside you and her legs are tucked under your arm. Continue to support your breast with a C hold using the opposite hand.

FIGURE 5-5:
Football hold

FIGURE 5-6:
Side-lying
position

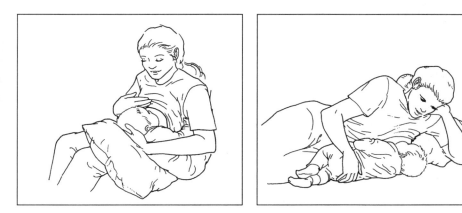

Side-Lying Position

Many women use the side-lying position to nurse their babies at night or if they are on bed rest for medical reasons. In this position, you can bring baby to bed with you and nurse while lying down. Both you and your baby lie on your sides facing each other, chest to breast. Baby is cradled in your arm with her head in the crook of your elbow. Her back is supported by the forearm on the same side you're nursing on. Baby's hip, shoulder and ear form a line. Use pillows to support your head, back and legs during this feeding. If you are anxious about trying this position at night, practise during the day until you feel more comfortable. Roll a towel or blanket to place behind your baby to support her back.

Over the Shoulder

If you have extremely large or heavy breasts, this position is the one that can sometimes save the breastfeeding relationship. Lie flat on your back on the floor or the bed. Position your baby over your shoulder so that she's lying tummy to shoulder with you. She is positioned face down over the nipple. You can monitor the latch from your position in the nosebleed section up above. If you have very large breasts and doubt your ability to perform these gymnastic feats, talk to a lactation consultant. She will guide you through the proper positioning to make breastfeeding successful.

If you are still pregnant and have a doll available, practise holding positions and the art of bringing baby to breast.

Using a variety of positions helps to work the breast from all angles and empties the breast more efficiently, reducing the risk of clogged ducts. With time, you and your baby will find a feeding pattern that works best. Perhaps you're right-handed and have found the cross-cradle position on the left breast most comfortable and the football hold on the right breast the best position.

Burping

Breastfed babies usually take in less air with their feedings than bottle-fed infants. But all babies need to be burped or they will cry when air bubbles sit in their stomachs. Here are a few of the most common methods of burping a baby.

Over-the-shoulder burping. Hold the baby against your chest with her head over your shoulder. Gently rub or pat her back until she burps.

Sitting-upright burping. Sit the baby on your knee and support her with the spread fingers of your hand on her chest. Use the web area of your hand to support her chin. The other hand supports her back as you gently pat her back to burp her.

Over-the-lap burping. Place baby on her tummy and across your lap. Pat or rub her back until she burps. Take care not to bounce your legs, as this will upset her stomach and she'll spit up on your feet.

FIGURE 5-7:
Over the
shoulder

FIGURE 5-8:
Sitting upright

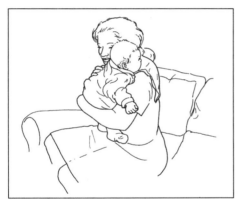

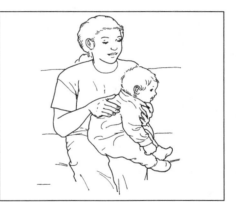

FIGURE 5-9:
Over the lap

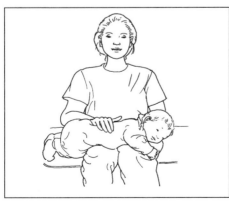

Burping should be slow and relatively gentle. You'll find that light patting and rubbing should produce the desired results within a few minutes. As with all the rest of the breastfeeding and burping routines, you will learn to understand what's 'normal' for your baby in time.

Spit-up

Although breastfed babies spit up less often than formula-fed infants, you can still expect to have a little of your breastmilk returned to you. Don't be alarmed if your baby occasionally spews. It may look as if she spits up her entire meal, but it's often not as much as it appears. Take a tablespoon of water and pour it on the kitchen worksurface. It might look like a lot, but considering your baby is taking in about 60g (2oz) at a single feeding, a tablespoon is a drop in the bucket. However, any projectile vomiting should be reported to your doctor.

Chapter 6

Fine-Tuning

J ust when you think you know so much, there are so many more things to consider. Breastfeeding is not just mealtime for your baby – it requires comfort, quiet and relaxation for both of you. Your location, routine and attitude all play a part in a positive and successful experience. Don't forget that in time, breastfeeding will become less complicated as you and baby find your groove.

Your Breastfeeding Environment

Comfort is the key to your breastfeeding environment. You'll want to set up a special place for your 'nursing nest'. Whether it's a favourite chair in a corner of your living room, a space in the baby's nursery, or even your bed, a relaxed and calm atmosphere makes the best nursing nest. The following are some ideas to consider when choosing your place:

Burping cloths – Keep your supply of burping cloths close by. You might use several at each feeding in the first few weeks, so have at least a dozen or so within easy reach of your chair or bed.

Chair – Whether it's a stuffed recliner, a decorative swing seat or a wooden rocking chair, your chair should be comfortable. You'll need support for your back and arms as well as your legs. You'll be using the chair for long periods of time throughout the day and night, so look for one that you like.

Climate – Your home should be kept at a temperature that's comfortable for everyone. Your nursing nest should be strategically placed away from draughts in the winter and hot or stuffy spots in the summer. Pay attention to the location of heating and cooling vents or radiators – the temperature near heating and cooling outlets varies a lot more than it does elsewhere in the room. Finally, keep a blanket handy for both of you.

Drink – Take one with you and keep it within easy reach. It's inevitable that you'll become thirsty when your baby starts to nurse.

Lighting – Try to pick a location that allows you to control the lighting; you'll want to keep the room dimly lit at night and at nap times. Bright lights don't seem to bother nursing babies, but they might make it more difficult for you to relax. A table lamp near your chair or bed is perfect. Windows should be curtained or shaded, both for light control and privacy. Avoid windows that face east: when the morning sun shines through the east windows at 6:00 AM, you and your baby might find it more difficult to go back to bed for that last stolen hour of sleep.

Magazine – Reading a magazine or a book while your baby nurses is a pleasant way to pass the time. You can keep up on world events, read about the joys of parenting, or just get lost for a while in a good novel. Breastfeeding gives you plenty of quiet, guilt-free reading time.

Music/TV – Listening to music or watching your favourite programmes can help you relax.

Pillows – You'll need pillows for support as well as to raise your lap.

Table – You'll need a table to hold your drink, remote control, book and perhaps a breast pump. A sturdy end table or a coffee table should work. You might want to have a phone handy, as well as the phone numbers of your health-care providers.

Just as with sitting down to do anything, getting settled to breastfeed will require a bit of planning and a bit of compromise. You'll forget the phone. Or the remote control. Or the nursing pillow. You'll know soon enough which accessories you can live without – and which are critical to your success.

Establishing a Routine

Newborn routine is an oxymoron. As days melt into nights and you walk in a twilight slumber, you'll wish your newborn knew what routine meant. But with the passing weeks, things will change and your baby will develop a fairly predictable schedule for eating, sleeping, playing and eliminating. You'll become more in tune with your infant's cues and able to anticipate what will follow next.

There is value in routines. They give adults some sense of control, and as children get older, routines promote good habits and give them a feeling of security and structure.

The Early Days

You might be waking your baby every two to three hours to feed, particularly in the first two weeks. You'll offer your baby your breast eight to 12 times in every 24-hour period. Demand feeding won't begin until after your sleepy baby has had time to regulate her internal body clock, about two to three weeks after birth. At that time, you'll breastfeed as often as your baby wants. It might be anywhere between one and four hours, or it might be a series of evening cluster feeds. Your baby will let you know when she's hungry. However, during those early sleepy days, you'll be waking her to ensure that she has plenty of opportunities to eat, drink and be merry.

Should I provide formula supplements during my baby's growth spurts?
Supplemental feedings of formula are unnecessary. Cluster feedings can be unnerving, but they are a natural way for your baby to stimulate increased milk production, and for your breasts to meet that demand for your growing infant.

At around three weeks of age, some babies want to nurse every hour, particularly if they are entering a growth spurt. These frequent nursings are called cluster or bunch feeds. Babies seem to space their feedings closer together at certain times of the day or night, then wait long periods between nursing sessions. It seems that just as you're ready to take your baby from the breast, she begins to root again. Cluster feeds are usually followed by longer periods of uninterrupted deep sleep, a sign that your baby is going through a growth spurt. Cluster feedings can cause a new mother to wonder if she's producing enough milk for her hungry baby. They can also try a mother's patience, but the phase is usually temporary (until the next time).

This is the way you will be developing your newborn 'routine' for the next couple of weeks:

You will watch your baby.	>	Your baby will give hunger cues.
You will position your baby, chest to chest.	>	Your baby takes position to nurse.
You prepare to latch baby to your breast.	>	Your baby latches on.
You drink according to thirst.	>	Your baby nurses to satiety.
You feel sleepy.	>	Your baby feels sleepy, too!

When your baby begins to doze or flutter suck after feeding for some time, burp her and offer her the second breast. Your baby will probably have a bowel movement once or twice during the nursing session. The nappy change can correspond with the breast switch.

Moving On

It might take up to three weeks before you learn to read your infant's cues well, but you will. Soon, you'll be expert at interpreting even her most subtle of cues, as only a parent can.

As your baby gets older, you'll begin to establish other routines as well. Your bedtime routine may include activities like a bath, a massage, a story, soft music or lullabies, rocking and a bedtime snack. Start bedtime routines early in life so your baby will begin to make associations between these transitions and sleep. But choose your bedtime routine carefully – you might not mind an hour-long process now, but in a few years it might lose some of its charm. Many of the bedtime routines you establish now will become steadfast habits when your baby grows into a toddler.

Your Baby's Sleep/Wake Cycle

Babies don't know whether it's day or night. They tell time, not by a clock or sundial, but by their own internal regulators. Infants move through predictable states of arousal every day. This is called the sleep/wake cycle, and it includes six states that your baby will move through in sequence.

State one. Quiet or deep sleep is characterized by little or no activity. You'll observe your baby's chest rising and falling rhythmically, a sign of deep relaxation. Your baby's eyelids will be closed, and she'll move very little. Babies in this state don't seem to have any awareness of light or sound. Every 30–45 minutes, she might move in a cycle between deep sleep and active sleep. When people say they sleep like a baby, this is what they mean!

State two. Active or light sleep is another sleep state. You'll see your baby's eyes darting around under her lids. This is called rapid eye movement (REM). You'll also notice her muscles twitching and facial expressions like smiling or frowning. Babies often make chewing motions or sucking sounds in light sleep.

State three. Drowsiness is a transitional state between sleep and waking. Babies have a dazed, unfocused, dreamy-eyed appearance while drowsy. Your baby's eyes might open and close, her breathing pattern is irregular, she might wake if stimulated and might exhibit a startled response to loud noises.

State four. The quiet alert state is the best time to breastfeed or perform infant massage. Babies are relaxed, alert, focused and observant, and they maintain good eye contact and have that 'lover's gaze'. Your baby is awake and ready for breakfast!

Even though your baby is small, it's important to change her positions and environment frequently throughout the day. Rocking, singing, talking, taking walks, massaging, playing on the floor and being carried by sling all help to offer opportunities for your baby to explore! Intelligence is built like a pyramid: the broader the base, the higher the peak.

State five. Active alert is the state where your baby is busy. She begins to vocalize or 'talk', she may become fussy, and her feet are constantly moving. She is easily overstimulated in this state, which can move her into the next: crying.

State six. Crying is a state, too. You'll know this one well after the first week. And after a while, you'll be able to distinguish between baby's cries of hunger, boredom, fatigue, pain, loneliness and overstimulation. Sometimes babies just need to blow off steam, and then they move the cycle back around to sleep.

Some babies make a transition smoothly from one state to the next, while others change so quickly you wonder whether they have a diagnosable personality disorder. Your baby's transitioning style is, in part, due to her individual personality and temperament.

In their first two weeks of life, babies eat and sleep, eat and sleep, eat and sleep. In their first week, they sleep for an average of 12–20 hours per day, and then the pattern changes, as shown below.

SLEEP CHART			
	DAY	**NIGHT**	**TOTAL**
First week	8–10	8–10	16–20
One month	7–10	7–8	14–18
Three months	6–8	6–8	12–16
Six months	4–6	6–8	10–14
Nine months	3–5	8–10	11–15
Twelve months	2–4	8–10	10–14

This sleep schedule indicates hours of sleep in a 24-hour period, not consecutive hours of sleep! If you manage to get four uninterrupted hours of sleep, count yourself lucky. Baby-care shifts work well during the early weeks, so both you and your partner have an opportunity to sleep undisturbed for a short period of time.

Night sleep patterns do not mean after midnight, either – 'night' is any time after the sun goes down. Sleep time will increase at night as your baby begins to have fewer naps.

Waking Your Sleepy Baby

Because babies spend their first two weeks in a sleepy state, they must be woken up every two to three hours for feeding. Remember that frequent feedings mean a more abundant milk supply for you and healthy weight gain for your baby.

Here is a bag of tricks to wake your sleepy baby for feeding:

- Change her nappy or gently wipe her face or back with a cool damp flannel.
- Gently stroke her mouth, cheeks and lips.

- Hold her skin-to-skin with you or Dad.
- Hold her upright under her arms and, while supporting her neck and head, gently bounce her, sing to her or offer her your clean finger to stimulate her sucking response.
- Lie her on her back and stimulate her skin with massage.
- Rub the palms of her hands and the soles of her feet.
- Try scalp massage by drawing small circles on her head with your fingers.
- Unswaddle your baby or remove her clothing.

You don't have to rouse her completely to a wide-awake state to nurse her, especially in the middle of the night. Keep the lights low and block out external noises that might startle her. She needs to be alert enough to nurse but not so much so that she has a hard time going back to sleep.

Middle-of-the-Night Feedings

Perhaps the biggest adjustment new parents must make is to their sleep schedule. Before your baby was born, you slept when you were tired and stayed in bed for as long as you wanted. Now the amount of sleep you get will depend on your baby.

Check your baby's sleeping environment for safety. Always place her on her back on a firm mattress. Don't use overstuffed blankets or duvets. Remove pillows and toys from your baby's crib. Keep the room temperature comfortable, neither hot nor cold. Dress baby for sleeping the same as you would dress yourself.

Your newborn doesn't have a set schedule, and even after he does, you'll be up several times in the night to feed him. The quality of your sleep will change: you'll sleep more lightly, almost with one eye open and one ear on the baby monitor. If you are sharing the bed, every little stir will rouse you.

You'll even develop a strategy with your spouse called the 'I'm Sleeping, It's Your Turn' game. Here's how to play: Your baby calls out, but both parents lie quietly, pretending to be asleep. The first one who moves, loses. Your internal dialogue goes something like this, 'Please, please get up. Can't you see I'm exhausted? I'm not moving. It's your turn. And if it's not your turn, it's still your turn! Get up!' Then, give your partner a subtle kick: 'You're it.'

If you're expressing milk, the diplomatic alternative is to simply swap nights or take shifts. You can work 10:00 PM to 2:00 AM, and he gets 2:00 AM to 6:00 AM.

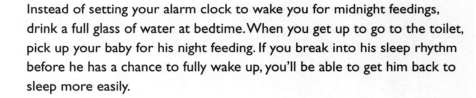

Instead of setting your alarm clock to wake you for midnight feedings, drink a full glass of water at bedtime. When you get up to go to the toilet, pick up your baby for his night feeding. If you break into his sleep rhythm before he has a chance to fully wake up, you'll be able to get him back to sleep more easily.

Most babies wake two to three times to be fed throughout the night. Some sleep in four-hour stretches. (Those probably belong to the same women who were never sick during pregnancy, had easy labours and now look as if they were never pregnant.) Keep external stimulation to a minimum, unless you're trying to wake a sleepy baby for a feeding.

At around six or seven months of age, or when solids are introduced, babies will often begin to sleep through the night. If they're offered a varied diet during the day, they might not need to feed at night as frequently as before. There's no hard and fast rule, though – your baby will let you know when he needs to nurse.

The Family Bed

Bedsharing has been a cultural practice for all but a few Western societies since the beginning of time. Japanese, Chinese, Indian and other cultures shared beds with newborns as a way to give babies shelter and security. Even in the UK and USA in times past, parents shared their beds with infants and toddlers – the author's grandfather slept at the foot of his parents' bed, along with other siblings, until he was six years of age. This was a custom of the times, one born out of need due to limited space, access to heat and family economics.

Popular Opinion

The idea of bedsharing has received mixed reviews from health-care providers, families and society in general. It isn't for everyone, but it does have some tremendous benefits for breastfeeding families.

Breastfeeding mothers feel more in sync with their bedsharing infants: they share the same sleep cycles, and mothers often report feeling more rested as a result. They approach nighttime feedings with a relaxed attitude. This ability to relax helps their milk ejection reflex work more effectively. Mothers simply gather their infants in their arms and side-lie as their babies nurse at the breast. Their babies often fall asleep again without completely entering an alert state.

Benefits for Baby

Studies have shown that babies who bedshare cry less than babies who sleep alone. They also gain weight more consistently. In fact, one of the methods prescribed by doctors who diagnose breastfeeding problems is for the mother to simply take her infant to bed, to rest and nurse.

The family bed might even help reduce your baby's risk of Sudden Infant Death Syndrome (SIDS). Bedsharing studies by Dr James McKenna indicate that infants sharing with their parents spend greater time in active or light sleep than infants who sleep alone. SIDS most often occurs when infants are in a state of deep sleep.

If you share with your baby, make sure your sleeping environment is as safe as her crib to prevent the risk of SIDS. Don't place babies on waterbeds, beanbag chairs or padded mattresses. Remove all pillows from around your infant, as well as blankets and duvets. Bedsharing by itself neither causes nor prevents SIDS.

Other doctors have strong feelings against bedsharing. They believe that this practice creates a dependent relationship in which children will have difficulty learning to calm themselves when they leave the family bed. Further, they believe it sets families up for sleep problems later in life.

Make an Informed Decision

It's important to remember when making choices about bedsharing that doctors are often offering their own personal opinions on this subject. They may not have studied this issue in medical school, and sometimes a doctor's opinion, like anyone's opinion, might have no basis in fact. Ask for current research on best practices, and remember that there are two sides to every issue. Most health-care providers remain flexible and offer bedsharing as an important option for breastfeeding pairs.

Don't introduce cereal or other solids early just to help your baby sleep through the night. Your baby's digestive system is not mature enough to handle those foods until around four to six months of age.

Talk to other families who have made this choice. Most importantly, talk to your spouse or bed partner. Men sometimes don't like sharing a bed with infants and toddlers; they might be afraid of rolling over onto the baby, or they might resent the loss of intimacy. It's also possible that a one-off swift kick in the wrong spot will leave your man sleeping in an uncomfortable defensive position.

Many men share a bed with their babies without problem or complaint, but that doesn't mean that a good father should necessarily be willing to sharing. Alternatives to cobedding include having a cradle at your bedside, purchasing a bedsharing bedding device or moving the baby's crib into your room. The crib mattress should be tight against your own mattress at the same level, without any space between the two. Lock or block the crib wheels to prevent a gap from forming between the mattresses. You might even consider tying the crib frame to your bed frame for a nice, secure fit. You can adjust the crib gate so you can easily pick up your infant for breastfeeding in the middle of the night.

Safety First

Dr William and Martha Sears state that parents instinctively know not to roll over on their babies. 'The same subconscious awareness that keeps you from rolling off the bed keeps you from rolling onto baby.' Still, there are precautions you should take.

Bedsharing does not have to affect your ability to engage in amorous adventures with your spouse. However, you might be inclined to discover new areas of the house. Changing times and places can add an element of surprise to your lovemaking that you both might find exciting.

Make sure that your bed is not overcrowded. Toddlers should not sleep with infants, as they thrash in their sleep, often turning sideways in bed without any conscious awareness of it.

Obviously, parents should not use any drugs or alcohol while bedsharing with their infants. The risk of suffocation is far greater when a parent is under the influence. And do not use duvets or heavy blankets.

Sudden Infant Death Syndrome

Sudden Infant Death Syndrome (SIDS) is the sudden and unexplainable death of infants from birth to one year of age. More boys than girls are victims, and most deaths happen during the autumn, winter, and early spring months.

Fortunately, the Foundation for the Study of Infant Death's (FSID) Back to Sleep Campaign is one that works. In the first year of the campaign, the number of babies dying of SIDS halved – that's an incredible number of lives saved through prevention.

To reduce the risk of SIDS (also known as cot death):

· Cut smoking in pregnancy – fathers too!
· Do not let anyone smoke in the same room as your baby.
· Place your baby on her back to sleep.
· Do not let your baby get too hot.
· Keep baby's head uncovered – place your baby with his head to the foot of the cot, to prevent wriggling down under the covers.
· Put your baby to sleep at night in your bedroom for the first six months.
· Avoid sharing your bed with a baby if you or your partner:
  – are smokers
  – have been drinking alcohol
  – take medication or drugs that make you feel drowsy – including any street drugs
· Do not sleep with your baby on a sofa or armchair.
· If your baby is unwell, seek medical advice promptly.

If your baby has a birth defect or has a breathing, heart or lung condition, or any other special need, talk to your health-care provider. While many mothers worry that infants might choke on their spit-up, research does not indicate this to be a threat. There is no increase in suffocation-related deaths because of back sleeping.

Do not smoke around your baby, and do not allow others to smoke around your baby. SIDS deaths are more common in families who smoke. In fact, the risks of smoking and bedsharing have been correlated with SIDS. Just as you wouldn't smoke in bed for your own health reasons, do not smoke in bed with your baby.

There are times when it's appropriate to place your baby on her stomach, but not at bedtime. Babies need opportunities for tummy time to help develop muscles and skills. When your baby is alert and you are with her, place her on her tummy. This is a great opportunity for infant exercise!

Make sure that your child-care provider, as well as your baby's alternative caregivers and grandparents, follow these important prevention strategies, too. Consistency in care is critical. Babies who are used to sleeping on their backs but are placed on their tummies in another's care are actually at 20 times greater risk of SIDS.

Soft mattresses and pillows pose a hazard because they can fold around your baby's mouth and nose. Avoid the use of frilly, overstuffed duvets, sheepskin, heavy fleeces and bumper pads in your baby's crib. If your baby is wearing a sleepsuit to bed, she needs only a light blanket. Similarly, don't place stuffed animals, toys or pillows in your baby's cradle. These, too, are suffocation hazards.

CHAPTER 7

Is This Right? Evaluating Breastfeeding

Most mothers are concerned that they might not have enough milk to nourish their infant. This is a common, but unnecessary, fear. Our uncertainty over our milk supply arises because we like to measure everything scientifically. When you breastfeed, there is no reliable direct method of knowing how much milk your baby receives, but doctors generally follow two guidelines when assessing breastmilk intake: infant weight gain and elimination patterns.

Weight Gain

Infant weight gain is one of the most important indicators of an adequate milk supply. However, it's normal for babies to lose 5–8 per cent of their birth weight during the first few days of life. After that, babies gain about 30g (1oz) of weight per day, and by their two-week check-up, they should surpass their birth weight by a few grams. Any baby who weighs less than her birth weight at her two-week checkup might not be feeding adequately.

All too often, parents are concerned when their infant is in the low or high end of the growth chart for their age. If you are checking against a centile chart, make sure that it is one designed for breastfed babies.

Breastfed babies gain weight more rapidly than formula-fed infants during the first two months of life, then slow down around the fourth month. By six months of age, their birth weight should have doubled. If you have concerns about your baby's weight, call your doctor. You can have your baby weighed at any time.

Elimination Patterns

The second-best indicator of adequate milk intake is frequent bowel movements and urination. What goes in must come out.

Soon after birth, your baby will pass meconium, a thick, sticky, dark substance produced by the liver. After two days, your baby's bowel movements will change to a greenish-brown colour and will look like thick pea soup. He will pass two to three stools per day. By day five, your baby's stools will change again, this time to a loose, mustard-yellow, cottage cheese or seed-like consistency. These are called milk stools. Your baby will pass two to five stools per day, most probably during a feeding, or when he's fast asleep and ready to be put down.

Your baby will also wet frequently. During the first two days, he might wet only once or twice. The colostrum you produce is highly digestible and perfect nutrition for your baby, so there's not much left to eliminate. After your abundant milk comes in, your baby will wet five to eight cloth nappies per day, or four to six disposables. With ultra-absorbant nappies on the market, it can be hard to tell how much he has wet. You can lay a Kleenex inside the nappy to help you tell when your baby urinates.

Call your doctor if your baby exhibits symptoms of dehydration: lethargy, weak cry, dry mouth, depressed or sunken fontanelle (soft spot) on the top of his head, loss of skin resilience (springiness) or fever.

The urine will be pale yellow or colourless and odourless. If it's dark or looks like red brickdust, it could be a sign that your baby is not getting enough milk. If your baby is wetting frequently but not stooling, he might not be getting enough hindmilk.

If your baby is not passing at least two stools per day and wetting six to eight nappies after his first week of life, he could be on his way to dehydration. This is a very serious health threat for babies, so talk to your doctor or health visitor immediately.

Breast Changes

Your breasts change during pregnancy, then once more with the birth of your baby, and again after a solid nursing routine is established. Lactogenesis leaves breasts full within three to five days postpartum.

Most women produce 30ml (1fl oz) of milk per breast per hour. Breasts generally feel full before a feeding and softer afterward, but because breasts don't have fuel gauges, the only sure way to measure your milk is to express it. Even then, you won't get a true indication of your milk volume, as a pump simply cannot remove milk as efficiently as your baby can.

According to infant studies, your baby needs about 30–60ml (1–2fl oz) of milk per feeding per month of age.

Day 1:   5ml/^{1}/$_6$fl oz (colostrum)
Day 2:   15ml/^{1}/$_2$fl oz (colostrum)
Day 3:   30ml/1fl oz (colostrum)
Day 4:   60ml/2fl oz (transitional milk)
Day 5:   60–75ml/2–2^1/$_2$fl oz (transitional milk)

You can also gauge how much your baby needs at each feeding by his weight:

170–225g (6–8lb):   60ml (2fl oz)
255–340g (9–12lb):   90ml (3fl oz)
367–425g (13–15lb):   125ml (4fl oz)
425+g (15+lb):   150ml (5fl oz)

As your baby suckles, you might feel a tingling or pins and needles sensation that lets you know your milk is letting down. As you nurse your baby, milk leaking from the opposite breast is also a sign that your milk has let down.

What effect, if any, will an epidural during labour have on milk production?
Epidurals used during labour and delivery cause overhydration of body tissues. Overhydration makes it difficult for hormones that stimulate the production of milk, such as prolactin, to reach breast cells across this lake of fluid. If you've had an epidural during labour, talk to a lactation consultant before hospital discharge.

Some women don't have these sensations, nor do they observe leakage. If you don't know if your milk has let down, you might need the assistance of your health visitor. Stress and fatigue can inhibit the milk ejection reflex, and this can ultimately reduce your milk supply.

Some mothers feel tenderness during their first week of breastfeeding. However, this discomfort usually subsides after the baby has latched on correctly. If you experience sore, cracked or blistered nipples, your baby is not latching on correctly and might not be adequately removing milk from the breast.

If you have not experienced any change in your breasts during pregnancy or after the birth of your baby, you'll need to have a breast exam performed by your doctor. A rare condition exists in a very few women that affects the growth of their mammary tissues. This underdevelopment inhibits milk production. Women who have had breast reduction surgery or a mastectomy are also at risk of insufficient milk production. If your doctor has determined that you are physically incapable of producing enough milk to nourish your baby, you will be asked to supplement with formula.

BREASTFEEDING EVALUATION CHECKLIST

Does your baby let you know he's hungry?	Yes	No
Do you position your baby chest to breast with you?	Yes	No
Does your baby open his mouth wide to attach?	Yes	No
Does your baby latch on effectively?	Yes	No
Are his lips flanged around your breast?	Yes	No
Does your baby create a tight seal around your breast?	Yes	No
Is your baby's suck rhythmic for five to 10 minutes?	Yes	No
Do you see your baby's ear wiggle while he's feeding?	Yes	No
Do you offer both breasts at each feeding?	Yes	No
Do you feel your milk ejection reflex?	Yes	No
Can you feel your uterus contract when nursing?	Yes	No
Are your breasts softer after each feeding?	Yes	No
Is your baby's hunger satisfied after nursing?	Yes	No
Is your baby gaining weight?	Yes	No
Is your baby passing loose/soft stools two to three times daily?	Yes	No
Is your baby wetting at least five to eight nappies five days after birth?	Yes	No

If you've answered no to any of these questions, ask your health visitor to observe your baby during a feeding session. Any problem corrected now will ensure a more successful breastfeeding experience.

Supplemental Feeding and Alternative Methods

If your doctor or lactation consultant determines that your baby isn't getting enough milk, they will work with you to increase your milk production. Increasing breastfeeding frequency, feeding from both breasts and expressing your breastmilk with a double pump can all increase your prolactin levels and help you produce a more abundant supply.

There may be situations that require you to use an alternative feeding method for a short time as you build your milk supply. With the goal of exclusive breastfeeding in mind, practise any of these methods cautiously and only under the guidance of a lactation consultant or paediatrician. Alternative feeding should be used on a temporary basis to correct breastfeeding problems. It's not usually a viable long-term solution, and it's important to get your baby back to the breast as soon as possible.

SUPPLEMENTAL FEEDING DEVICES AND TECHNIQUES

Type	Description	Comments
Cup feeding	A flexible 30g (1fl oz) or60ml (2fl oz) cup is filled with milk and held to baby's lips. The baby is held upright and allowed to lick at the milk.	DO NOT POUR. Baby should not be crying at start.
Spoon feeding	This method is similar to cup feeding but utilizes a spoon. A small, soft spoon is best. Some special spoons hold larger amounts of milk in a reservoir so feeding isn't interrupted.	Tedious and time-consuming but effective.
Syringe/eyedropper feeding	An eyedropper can be used to drip milk into an upright baby's mouth. A syringe can be used in the same way. A syringe with a long tip can be used to feed at the breast.	Periodontal syringes are best; they have a soft tip that won't hurt baby's gums.
Finger feeding	The tube of a supplemental feeder is held to a clean adult finger. Baby sucks on the finger and gets milk through the tube.	Effective, but some babies prefer it to the breast.

(continued) |

TYPE	DESCRIPTION	COMMENTS
Standard bottle	Any variety of the plain old infant bottle.	Leads to nipple confusion and poor suck.

Cup or Spoon Feeding

Supplemental feeding using a cup can be beneficial for a baby who has jaundice, poor elimination patterns or inadequate latch. Cup feeding reduces nipple confusion from a bottle and allows the infant to lap milk at his own pace. Although cup feeding can be messy, it's an easy substitute for breastfeeding.

To begin, place a towel around your baby or swaddle him in a blanket. Fill a spoon or a soft, flexible cup half-full with expressed milk. Bring the cup or spoon to the baby's lower lip. Drip just enough milk into his mouth to taste. Tip the spoon so your baby can lick the milk. This process is slower than putting baby to the breast but can be used to supplement breastfeeding, as needed. The use of an eyedropper can also be effective.

Finger Feeding

Finger feeding is hard to learn, awkward and can cause dependency, but it is useful for babies who have a weak suck, nipple confusion or neurological problems.

Insert a small gavage tube into the nipple of a baby bottle filled with expressed milk. Place your baby in a semi-reclining position. Offer a clean finger (nail side down) slowly into your baby's mouth, moving it back to the soft palate. If your baby gags, bring your finger forwards slightly, and wait until he's comfortable. Place the tube or periodontal syringe next to your finger. As your baby suckles, he will draw milk from the bottle, or you can offer a small squirt from the syringe.

FIGURE 7-2:
Finger feeding

FIGURE 7-3:
Syringe feeding

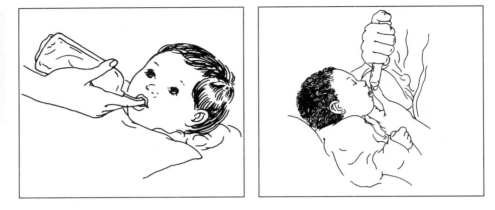

Bottle Feeding

Bottle feeding may be the only alternative available when other techniques don't work. It can be useful for mothers with sore nipples or if an infant can't open his mouth wide enough to latch to the breast. However, many babies who switch from breast to bottle and back again can suffer from nipple confusion – in addition, bottle nipples flow faster than the breast, and once babies develop a dependency on the bottle, they frequently refuse the breast.

Many parents find that infants accept supplemental feedings more easily from Dad than from Mum. A baby grows comfortable with the breastfeeding relationship she establishes with her mother and can sometimes be confused when her breastfeeding buddy tries to offer a less satisfying alternative.

Supplemental and alternative feeding methods give Dad a wonderful opportunity to take part in the feeding of his child. Finger feeding, cup feeding, spoons, bottles and eyedroppers can be used by anyone. Many fathers enjoy being able to solve problems, and giving supplemental feedings can be a rewarding way to help them feel more connected to their children.

CHAPTER 8

Common Concerns

Sometimes there are challenges when you're breastfeeding. Whether your baby has difficulty latching on or you need to suspend breastfeeding for your own health reasons, anything that interferes with milk removal can diminish your supply. If your baby doesn't take in enough milk, your body won't produce enough milk. Fortunately, most breast-feeding problems are easily resolved if you catch them early enough.

Does Breastfeeding Hurt?

You may experience some temporary discomfort during the first week of breastfeeding. Your baby takes your nipple and part of the areola to the back of his mouth, and he compresses the areola to express milk from the sinuses. You should feel a gentle tug that will take some getting used to.

If you do feel actual nipple pain while nursing, your baby might not be positioned correctly. Your nipple has more pain receptors than your areola, so, if your baby is feeding from the nipple, you'll feel it. Continued nipple feeding can lead to cracked or blistered nipples. Break the latch and try again. If everything else seems to be all right but nipple pain persists after a week, check for thrush.

Prolonged nipple pain is an indication that something is wrong. Contact your health visitor straight away if you experience any kind of pain while nursing your baby.

You may feel some minor breast discomfort with your milk ejection reflex or letdown. Sensations vary from slight tingles to pins and needles. Letdown lasts less than 30 seconds. You'll also feel some breast fullness with engorgement, but this normally decreases within two days.

Engorgement

Engorgement usually happens around three to five days post partum. Your mature milk comes in, in preparation for exclusive breastfeeding. When engorgement happens, it can be extremely uncomfortable. You wake up one morning with breasts the size of melons: they're swollen, your nipple and areola are tight, and your baby has little flexible tissue to latch onto. While this lasts only for a couple of days, it can be painful.

Frequent feedings will help reduce engorgement. They will also regulate your milk supply. If your baby has difficulty latching on, express just enough milk to make yourself comfortable and your breasts pliable.

After your baby has had her fill, you can express more milk and either refrigerate or freeze it for later use. (Remember, though, that any milk that is removed will be replaced. That's the law of supply and demand.)

Warm showers will relieve the pressure of engorgement, and your milk will begin to leak naturally. Heat, in general, will soften your breasts. A warm flannel on full breasts can help to alleviate discomfort.

Cabbage Leaves

Although there is no known medical reason why cabbage leaves should help with engorgement, many mothers and lactation professionals will attest to the fact that they work. Cabbage leaves have been used throughout the centuries in other countries. It's a timeless method of reducing engorgement.

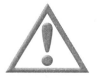

Cabbage leaves should be used only as long as the discomfort of engorgement lasts. Prolonged use can diminish your milk supply.

Here's what you do: buy a medium-size cabbage. Peel and clean the leaves, then store them in sealed plastic bags. Refrigerate. When you're ready to use them, select enough leaves to cover your breasts completely on all sides, as well as the area under your armpit. Gently crush the leaves to break the veins, then apply the cool leaves to your breasts. Lie back on a towel and relax, or tuck them securely into your bra. The cool cabbage leaves will help reduce the pain and swelling associated with engorgement.

Within two hours, you'll begin to feel relief. Some milk might leak, so if you're using the bra method, line your bra with nursing pads or other absorbent materials. You should reapply new leaves after two hours, or whenever they appear wilted.

Other Comfort Measures

Although the engorgement phase is relatively brief, you'll want to give yourself every advantage to ensure your comfort until your nursing routine is established. In addition to cool cabbage leaves and warm showers, consider the following suggestions:

·   Wear a supportive bra.
·   Take ibuprofen for pain.
·   Wrap a plastic bag of ice cubes or frozen vegetables in a tea towel or large flannel. (Peas or sweetcorn work best because of their size, but you can use whatever is available.) The bag will conform to the shape of your breast and can be used for 15–20 minutes of relief. If you plan to refreeze the bag of vegetables and use it again later, mark it as inedible – repeated freezing and thawing promotes the growth of bacteria.
·   A refrigerated rice sock works wonders, too. Rice socks are used by doulas to relieve pain during labour. They conform to your body and provide relief by interrupting the pain receptors that carry messages to the brain. Rice socks can be heated or cooled. To cool a sock, put it in the freezer for an hour. To heat, cook it in the microwave for 30 seconds at a time (for up to two minutes). When using the microwave method, carefully shake the sock so the heat is evenly distributed. Wrap the rice sock in a tea towel or sheet to protect your skin.

To make your own rice sock, fill a clean cotton tube sock with plain white rice. Add a drop of your favourite aromatherapy scent, such as lavender, for relaxation. Sew the top closed with a needle and thread. Rice socks can be used over and over again, but they cannot be washed. They last a long time and can be used to relieve aches and pains in daily life such as sore muscles, headaches and cramp.

Remember that this stage is only temporary. Try any combination of the relief methods until the discomfort passes and you and your baby can have a comfortable breastfeeding session.

Leaking

Many women have concerns that their milk will leak during business presentations or while out in public. This can happen. However, some women don't experience any leaking at all. Leaking most often occurs during the first few weeks of lactation, and usually only continues with women who have a very abundant milk supply. There are exceptions, of course, and leaking or even spraying milk during love-making is a relatively common occurrence.

If you experience frequent leaking:

· Nurse your baby frequently, especially before going out or making love.
· Use absorbent cotton breastpads or cloths to catch the drips.
· Place bath towels under you when in bed.
· Press your folded arms gently against your chest to draw your breasts into your body.

There are occasions when you'll experience letdown at the thought or smell of your baby. A crying child in the supermarket might even turn on your milk like a tap. Generally, however, most women who feed their babies regularly won't leak after a breastfeeding routine has become quite well established.

Sore Nipples and Blisters

Sore nipples are usually a sign of nipple feeding or improper latch. When babies feed only on the nipple, nipples can crack and blister. Blisters also occur as a result of rubbing against the roof of baby's mouth or along his gums. The pain associated with a blistered nipple can make nursing very uncomfortable, but it's important to continue breastfeeding.

Sometimes cracked nipples bleed, but that doesn't have to interfere with nursing. A little bit of your blood, mixed with your milk, will not harm your baby.

To treat sore nipples:

· Ensure that your baby has a good latch. (Wait until he opens wide, then grasp him to the breast, pointing your nipple to the roof of his mouth. He needs to take in 2.5cm/1in of the areola as well.)
· Use different nursing positions to vary the way your baby latches onto your nipple.
· Offer the least tender breast first so that your milk will let down in the other breast without your baby creating suction.
· Express your milk using a pump to help your milk let down before offering your breast to your baby.
· Break suction evenly by inserting your finger into your baby's mouth. (Don't allow your baby to slide off your nipple.)
· Apply lanolin to a sore nipple. (Like chapped lips, nipples heal more quickly with moisture. You don't need to remove modified lanolin before your baby nurses.)
· Use breast shells to keep your nipples from rubbing against fabric.

Remember, also, to avoid using soap on your nipples. The Montgomery glands produce natural oils to clean and protect your nipples; soap may aggravate the situation by drying them out further.

Clogged Ducts

Clogged milk ducts occur when there is an insufficient removal of milk from the breast. The retained milk forms a cheeselike blockage in the duct, causing a small lump that might be painful, red or swollen. If neglected, clogged ducts can lead to infections.

The best way to prevent a clogged duct is simply to breastfeed as often as your baby wants, making sure that he finishes one breast before starting another. It's also helpful to change nursing positions. Different positions help your baby remove the milk from all of the ducts. Finally, be sure to wear a comfortable bra. Avoid anything that binds or constrains the breasts, including underwires.

If one of your ducts does become clogged, check for a clogged nipple. Milk residue can sometimes dry in a nipple pore, forming a blockage. If you see a small white dot, like a whitehead, on your nipple, you might have a clogged pore. Nipple blockages are often removed by your baby's suckling. They can also be removed by your health-care provider, although many women find that careful work with a fingernail can do the trick.

If no nipple blockage is apparent:

· Apply a warm cloth to the affected area for 15–20 minutes before each feeding.
· Nurse more frequently, beginning each breastfeeding session with the affected breast.
· Massage the breast near the clogged duct as your baby nurses or in a warm shower, gently working from behind the plug towards the nipple.

When the clogging breaks loose, you might see a filament of solidified milk that looks like a string and can be several centimetres in length. If you see one of these strings in your baby's mouth after nursing, don't be alarmed. It's soft and safe to eat, and it won't choke your baby.

Mastitis

Mastitis is the word doctors use to describe an infection of the breast. These sorts of bacterial infections generally begin with a clogged duct or a cracked nipple. A mother with mastitis usually has flu-like symptoms along with a fever, and a hard spot or lump in the breast accompanied by pain, redness and swelling. Mastitis is often treated with antibiotics. Other measures include warm showers, lots of bed rest and fluids, and frequent nursing. The infection is not harmful to babies and is only aggravated by weaning.

Any time mastitis symptoms last beyond two days or a breast lump remains, you should suspect an abscess. A breast abscess is a pool of pus within the breast tissue. The fluid must be drained by your doctor.

Recovery is rapid after draining, but temporary weaning from the infected breast may be required.

Thrush

Thrush or candida is another name for a common yeast infection of both mothers and babies. Most children with candida became infected as they passed through the birth canal. The first symptoms usually occur in two to four weeks. On occasion, babies become infected much later, usually after the use of antibiotics. If you've nursed comfortably for many weeks or months but are suddenly experiencing pain, thrush may be the problem.

Infants with thrush have white patches inside their mouths or an angry rash on their bottoms. Mothers often have sharp, shooting pains in their breasts, and sometimes red, tender nipples or patches of red or white on the breast.

Thrush can be very painful, but it responds well to treatment. Doctors typically prescribe an antifungal rinse for the baby's mouth and an antifungal cream or ointment for the baby's bottom (boy or girl) and mother's nipples. However, medication alone is not always effective. In addition to medical treatment, you should:

- Rinse the affected breasts and nappy area with clean water and let them air-dry.
- Expose the affected area to the sun for a few minutes, once or twice per day.
- Change your nursing pads after every feeding session.
- Change nappies frequently – yeast thrives in warm, damp places.
- Wash bras, bottle nipples, breast shells, dummies and any other items that come into contact with the infected areas in hot, soapy water.
- Use lanolin or other breastfeeding-friendly nipple treatments to relieve pain.
- Wash your hands before and after each feeding or treatment.
- Drink more water and eat less sugar.
- Treat your partner if he has had contact with your breasts.

Many mothers successfully treat thrush with a non-prescription medication called gentian violet. Most pharmacies carry a 1 per cent solution of gentian violet that can be applied to all infected areas with a cotton swab, twice daily for three days. It's a pretty colour, but it stains everything it comes in contact with, so be careful with your clothing.

If you are expressing milk while you have a yeast infection, 'pump and dump': freezing does not kill yeast, and stored milk can reinfect your baby.

Nipple Confusion

If your baby has been fed from a bottle, he might find it difficult to feed from the breast. Similarly, a baby who's been exclusively breastfed can find the transition to a bottle difficult. Feeding from a bottle is different from breastfeeding: the suck is different. The volume and flow of milk are different. The taste, texture and temperature are different. Perhaps most importantly, bottles reward lazy nursing and breasts don't.

When your baby doesn't know how to suckle the breast properly because of bottle or dummy use, it's called nipple confusion. Nipple confusion threatens your breastfeeding success by compromising your milk production. Your infant's disorganized suck won't effectively remove the milk from your breast. That leads to a decreased milk supply, which leads many women to supplement nursings with a bottle of formula. However, you need a hungry baby's eager suckling to maintain your milk production.

tips

Because nipple confusion impairs breastfeeding success, new mothers should avoid giving their infants bottles or dummies for at least the first six weeks of life.

Whether you're changing your child from breast to bottle or bottle to breast, be patient and persistent. Your baby will make the change, but it may not happen on the first attempt. The best time to try a new feeding method is when your baby is awake and alert but not too hungry. Your baby will only be frustrated by the change if he's already fussing for dinner. The quiet-alert stage right after he wakes is best.

If you're going from bottle to breast, express some milk before you begin to trigger your letdown reflex. Babies who are used to bottles want their milk immediately. After your baby has caught on to breastfeeding, you can continue nursing him without any special preparation.

If you're making the transition from breast to bottle, you may need to experiment with a number of different nipple styles and materials to find one your child likes (see Chapter 13). There are quite a few varieties available, and babies definitely do have individual preferences. Start the move to bottle feeding with expressed breastmilk, but let Dad or another caregiver do the feeding. Some babies simply refuse to take a bottle from Mum when they know there's a perfectly good breast available.

Breastmilk Jaundice

Newborn jaundice is caused by the normal breakdown of excessive red blood cells into bilirubin, a substance that turns babies' tissues yellow. Breastmilk jaundice is different from other jaundice in that it usually occurs in well-fed babies who are older than seven days, and it can persist for many weeks. Some doctors believe that breastmilk contains an unknown substance that lets babies absorb an excessive amount of bilirubin, but don't let that theory scare you.

There is nothing wrong with your milk. The usual course of treatment is to monitor your baby's blood and wait for this normal, physiological process to end. Nurse often. Your baby's body eliminates bilirubin through her stools. The greater the frequency of bowel movements, the quicker the excess bilirubin leaves the body.

What can you do to preserve your milk supply while using alternate feeding methods?
Pump your breasts frequently to maintain your milk supply while your baby is taking formula. Ask about finger feeding or other methods to help reduce nipple confusion while your baby takes formula.

Occasionally, doctors recommend that a child be given formula instead of breastmilk for 12–24 hours. This quickly lowers the bilirubin levels in baby's bloodstream. However, even one day of bottle feeding can interfere with your breastfeeding success.

Teething and Biting

If and when your baby bites your nipple (and after you've regained consciousness), firmly tell her 'No' and break the latch. Look her in the eye and tell her 'No biting'. Be serious but not angry. She may already be in tears after your surprised reaction. Offer the breast again, but if she continues to bite, give her a teething toy to help reinforce its use. Offer expressed milk, water or juice in a baby cup to complete the feeding, and try breastfeeding again later. Soon your baby will begin to associate biting with the items you have offered, but your consistency is the key.

Do not offer a teething infant anything chokeable to help teeth erupt. Ice cubes and many frozen foods can easily lead to tragedy. Raw vegetables and hard fruits will have to wait until baby has lots of teeth with which to chew them.

Luckily, teething begins at around six months of age (depending in part on heredity), so most babies will be beginning solids. However, some babies are born with a tooth, so learning to get around this little dental ditty happens much earlier.

What if your baby refuses the breast because of teething pain? Again, try the cup. Or talk to your doctor or health visitor about using an over-the-counter infant teething gel. Your little darling might accept the breast more readily if her gums are numbed. You want to ensure that she's receiving adequate nutrition, so offer baby rice, expressed breastmilk or cold, 100 per cent natural, unsweetened apple sauce.

A Teething Primer

You won't find any hard and fast rules on how long it takes a baby to cut his teeth. Every baby is unique and tooth development happens at different rates, but it generally takes two weeks to two months once the tooth is near the surface of the swollen gum.

The pressure of biting helps relieve the pain of teething. Your baby is not being mean when he bites you; he is just doing what comes naturally. As you begin to notice signs that your baby is teething, develop a strategy. Offer him cooled teething rings; a wet, cool flannel; a feeding spoon; a baby cup lid; or a dummy. Cold will help numb his gums, while biting works the teeth through the gums.

Teething and Nipple Care

On occasion, a baby may break the skin on his mother's nipple with a bite. More commonly, teething will chap the nipple due to increased acids in the saliva or as a result of baby's teeth rubbing against the nipple. Use your breastmilk to coat the nipple and let it air dry. If your injury is severe, your doctor will recommend a safe antibiotic ointment for use between nursing sessions so bacteria doesn't cause infection. This will need to be washed off before you nurse your baby. Moist healing is preferred for nipple care and treatment.

Lack of Support

Many new mothers are understandably nervous about breastfeeding their babies. You've probably heard stories from family or friends who tried to breastfeed their babies but gave up. 'I couldn't produce enough milk' is the most common reason women give for abandoning nursing in favour of bottle feeding.

Often, the real cause in these cases was a lack of confidence and support. New mothers who aren't sure their baby is getting enough milk through nursing might be tempted to use formula. However, your breasts make only enough milk to supply your baby's demands. If you worry that you're not producing enough milk and offer formula, the amount of milk you produce decreases from a lack of demand. Then, you're in a downwards spiral. Less milk means more formula, which means less demand until pretty soon you've shut down altogether – all from lack of confidence.

Reassure bottle-feeding mums that they are good mothers, but if nothing works with the critics, surround yourself with positive voices instead. Get together with women who nursed successfully or join a lactation support group such as the La Leche League. Remember, you can do it!

A good lactation consultant, health visitor or doctor can help you be successful. So can your partner, family and friends. Unfortunately, there will be people who aren't supportive of your decision to breastfeed, and they can undermine your breastfeeding experience. Sometimes partners aren't too thrilled about sharing your breasts with a baby. Even other women might be defensive about your decision to breastfeed, especially if they bottle fed their own children – and this might include your own mother or mother-in-law. When you talk about the virtues of breastfeeding, they might feel a need to justify bottle feeding. Try to keep their fears in mind when they criticize your decision to nurse.

CHAPTER 9
Colic

Breastmilk is the best food for your child, and breastfeeding is the most comforting way in which she can get it. Still, colic can threaten your breastfeeding experience. Feelings of frustration and disappointment don't exactly leave you wanting to be close to your baby, much less nurse her, but there are things you can do to get through the experience and come out of it as a strong breastfeeding pair.

What Is Colic?

Crying is a very powerful tool! It is your baby's most effective means of communication. Babies cry for many different reasons. They cry when they're hungry. They cry when they're wet or have a dirty nappy. They cry when they feel scared, lonely or hurt. They even cry when they're bored. Within the first two weeks of your baby's life, you will learn to distinguish between your baby's different cries. You'll even be able to distinguish her cries from others in a roomful of babies!

Whenever your child cries, you know something is wrong and you instinctively come to her aid. Usually, you can find the problem quickly. You pick up your baby, check her nappy, reassure her and perhaps offer her a breast. When nothing seems to work, lay people will call it colic. Paediatricians are a little more precise, but not much. They usually consider a baby to be colicky if she follows the rule of three: she cries continuously for three or more hours, three or more times each week, for three or more weeks.

Between 10 per cent and 15 per cent of newborns suffer from colic. Symptoms usually begin within a few weeks of birth and last from three to four months. There are many theories, but no general agreement as to its cause.

'Colic' is a term used to describe inconsolable crying that can last for several hours, and is more prevalent in the evenings. Babies cry miserably and appear to be in pain, often drawing their knees up to their bodies and screwing up their faces, going red in the face and clenching their fists. Colic usually starts at around three to four weeks of age and peaks at about six to eight weeks. The condition normally stops by the time your baby is three months old, although some babies can continue to have 'colicky' symptoms for a number of months after this – these do also tail off, however.

Fretfulness versus Colic

It's important not to confuse colic with ordinary fretfulness. Crying infants are difficult to feed and do not breastfeed effectively. Fretful infants can be consoled at the breast. Most colicky infants cannot.

Every baby will have periods of fretfulness, especially during the first few weeks of life. Not only are they new to the world, but the world is new to them. It's louder, colder and brighter than the womb, and it can take some getting used to.

Is there a way to differentiate between colic and fretfulness?
Standard fretfulness seems to follow predictable patterns. Crying often peaks with babies in their second week of life. They cry more frequently and with more intensity because of environmental overstimulation and growth spurts.

Just like adults, every baby has a different temperament, and some are naturally more demanding and sensitive than others. Think of these high-maintenance babies as having especially sharp senses. Windy pain that wouldn't upset most babies can be very distressing to one with more delicate sensibilities.

Growth Spurts and Temperament

Babies experience growth spurts around two to three weeks and again at six weeks. During these times, your baby might be fretful because she is hungry. You're making enough milk, it's just time to take production up another notch. Your baby is growing and preparing your body for the additional nourishment she needs.

Babies experiencing growth spurts tend to feed more often, especially during the evening. After several cluster feeds, your baby will doze off for several hours. Because your milk supply is lower in the evening, your baby can cluster feed without developing gastritis.

Letting your baby nurse more often will quickly increase your milk supply and satisfy her appetite. If you are returning to work during this time, frequent pumping is important.

What Causes Colic?

The cause of colic is unknown. Experts believe that colic may be a more extreme form of normal crying, but it could also be caused by a disturbance in your baby's immature immune system. If your baby is crying inconsolably, consult your doctor to rule out the possibility that your baby is ill.

If your baby makes frequent clicking or slurping sounds at the breast, suspect a poor seal between the breast and her mouth, or that her tongue is out of position. Poor latch will allow your baby to swallow air, increasing the chances of an upset stomach and wind pains.

What Can I Do?

Your baby will not develop colic because of anything you do or fail to do. Some parents find the following methods helpful, but be careful not to overstimulate your baby.

- Give your baby a warm bath.
- Swaddle him so he feels secure.
- Massage her feet.
- Let him suck a dummy.
- Use colic drops or gripe water as directed.
- Try cranial osteopathy from a qualified practitioner.

Ask your health visitor or a breastfeeding counsellor for advice. Although it is distressing, colic will cause no lasting damage to your baby's health.

Sound

Your vacuum cleaner is about to become your new best friend. The sound of a vacuum has been known to calm a colicky baby instantly. Get out the Hoover and give it a try. If you can't use the vacuum cleaner, tune the television to a static-filled channel and turn up the volume. Other good sources of white noise are detuned radios or small appliances such as blenders, mixers and tumble dryers. You can even buy the sounds of your child's favourite appliances on tape or CD for use away from the home.

Another calming sound for many babies is music. It's certainly worth a try for your colicky baby. If you played a particular piece of music during pregnancy or you often sing to your child, those songs might help her relax. If not, experiment with different types of music. The one that works might not be your favourite style, but you'll soon learn to love it out of sheer gratitude.

f@ct

You might be tempted to just forget about breastfeeding and switch to formula, but that can be a major mistake. Most babies who have a food allergy are sensitive to cows' milk, the primary ingredient in baby formula. Instead of eliminating colic, formula may actually make it worse.

Don't underestimate the power of your own voice cooing softly in your baby's ear. Use your voice as an instrument. Sing. Change tones. Babies respond well to 'parentese', that higher-pitched tone that mums and dads often use when speaking to infants.

Movement

Movement is soothing to all babies. Anyone who has ever cared for a crying child knows that rocking, bouncing or the gentle vibrations of a moving vehicle can lull a baby into sleep. Calming movement seems instinctive when you try to soothe your child. Most parents have tried rocking and gently bouncing their baby in their arms, but don't stop there. Try dancing, moving from side to side, baby swings and bouncy chairs. Movement is often more effective when combined with some of the other techniques. Placing your baby in her car seat on top of a running clothes dryer provides gentle movement and white noise at the same time. (If you do try this, make sure both your baby and her seat are secure.)

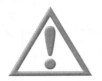

Never shake your baby! Shaken baby syndrome has claimed the lives of countless newborns. Colic is frustrating for both parent and infant. If you feel like you're on your last nerve, call a friend, family member, health visitor or crisis line immediately.

Some movements help your baby expel painful gas. Try putting gentle pressure on your infant's tummy, or try the colic hold. Put your baby face-down along the length of your arm: her head goes off to one side of your arm at the inner bend of the elbow, her arms and legs dangle on either side of your forearm, and your hand cups her bottom. Your other hand can then rub her back as you walk or bop in place. This hold takes a lot of strength, so it can be a good reason to hand your crying baby to your partner for a while.

FIGURE 9-1:
Colic hold

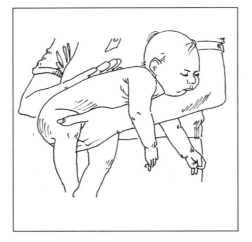

The colic hold places gentle pressure on your baby's tummy, which may ease digestive pains. Combine this hold with rhythmic motions and soothing sounds to help keep you and your baby calm.

A variation on the colic hold turns the baby around on your arm (with her head towards your palm) and lets your other arm come up underneath to help support the baby's weight.

Warm Bath

Some parents have found that taking a colicky baby into a tub of warm water will calm her. This is not only great therapy for your child, it's wonderfully relaxing for you. At the first sign of colic, you both get into the bath and stay there. You might be there all morning or half the night – just keep adding warm water along the way and nursing when you need to. Lie your baby on your chest, tuck her knees to her tummy and cover her with a warm flannel. Gently and continuously cup warm water over her back. The moist heat and skin-to-skin contact have been known to work wonders. Washing your baby with a gentle, scented cleanser enhances the relaxing effects of the bath with a combination of aromatherapy and massage. Lavender is a calming scent for both of you.

 Although a warm bath can provide a welcome break from the symptoms of colic for your baby, parents need to take extreme caution with this approach. A tired mum or dad in the bath can easily fall asleep, and an infant could drown.

The use of aromatherapy in childhood can lead to a lifetime of relaxation. Nothing brings back a memory like the smells associated with an event. Think about your grandmother's kitchen or the smell of a new on Christmas morning. The soft sweetness of the lavender that calms your colicky child now will probably become associated with a feeling of relief and relaxation for the rest of her life.

Swaddling

Swaddling is a way of snugly wrapping your infant in a blanket. This technique sometimes helps to calm a colicky baby. Swaddling keeps her warm and secure, like a cloth hug. It's also a way to keep her from being upset by the way her own body suddenly jerks when she's startled. Swaddled babies often sleep longer and are less fretful.

During early infancy, most babies are swaddled from the neck down. Your baby might prefer to have her arms free. Try it both ways. Older babies, however, are generally frustrated by swaddling. If your child is learning to roll or crawl, it's probably time to stop.

Slings

Slings have been used for centuries by mothers in many cultures to keep their babies close to their bodies for warmth, protection and transportation. Slings act as 'transitional wombs'. Your baby is close to your breast, can hear your heartbeat, and grows in sync with your body rhythms. Dads who carry their babies in slings bond more quickly as both learn to read each other's cues and movements. Babywearing meets an infant's need for sensory stimulation. Constant contact with their caregivers promotes happier, healthier babies, and studies indicate that sling-carried infants cry less frequently than other babies.

Infant Massage

Massage can often bring a measure of relief to a colicky baby. It can help your baby's body release trapped wind by pushing wind and faecal matter through the intestines to the bowel. Massage also promotes the normal functioning of the intestines, stimulates nervous system development and provides an opportunity for mother and child to work together in a relaxing and bonding way.

The specific techniques used to massage a colicky baby tend to focus on the abdominal area. Try this:

1. Find a warm, quiet place.
2. Sit on the floor with your back straight and your legs in front of you. Your knees should be bent out to the sides, and your heels should touch.
3. Place your baby on a soft blanket on the floor within the area between your legs.
4. Relax.
5. Ask your baby if she wants a massage. This will serve as her cue that you're about to begin.
6. Remove baby's clothes and nappy. Talk about what you're doing.

7. Stroke gently with your hands, palm down on baby's stomach, one hand after the other.
8. Hold your baby's legs up by the ankles with your left hand and continue using scooping strokes on her stomach with your right hand.
9. Put baby's legs down and lie your thumbs flat at her navel. Push out to the sides with the flats of your thumbs. Don't poke.
10. Repeat steps 7 to 9 six times.
11. Hold your baby's knees together and gently but firmly push them into her stomach. Hold them there for 30 seconds.
12. Gently release your baby's legs and put both hands, palm down, on her stomach. Your right hand should be above your left hand.
13. As your left hand makes a circle moving clockwise, your right hand makes a half-circle in the same direction. A clockwise motion is important because that's the direction food and wind flow in the intestines.
14. Repeat steps 12 to 13 six times, followed again by step 11.

When massaging your baby, use a light natural oil (such as vegetable oil), not lotion. Baby oil has petroleum products that can seep into baby's skin. Keep all of your motions gentle, long, slow and rhythmic.

Continue Nursing

Your milk is giving your baby everything she needs to get through this difficult time. As a nursing mother, it might comfort you to know that you can offer your baby a few moments of relief at your breast. If at some point you feel that you just can't do it anymore, express your milk and bottle feed it to your baby.

Coping with a Colicky Infant

The stress caused by a screaming baby, combined with a new parent's lack of confidence and lack of sleep, can take a huge toll on your health and self-esteem. A baby with colic puts a tremendous strain on a family, especially on a nursing mother. It's not uncommon for women to feel disappointed and even angry about their colicky child. Remember that it's not your baby's fault. She's not crying because she is 'spoiled' – she's simply in pain. There's no such thing as a spoiled infant.

Many colicky babies have their crying jags in the evening when you're already worn out from the day's activities, so sleep whenever you can – always good advice to new parents, this is incredibly important for parents of a colicky baby. One of you can take the baby to a far corner of the house or on a long drive while the other naps. Fathers need to step up during colic attacks and offer relief to their breastfeeding partners whenever they can.

A colicky baby does not make you a bad parent. It also doesn't mean there's anything wrong with your breastmilk or your genetics. There seems to be no common thread connecting colicky infants, not birth order, culture, class, gender or anything that happened during pregnancy or birth. Colic just happens.

In time, the screaming and crying can really wear you and your partner down and deflate your excitement about being parents. Every expectant couple has a dream about what it's going to be like when the baby finally arrives: we all envision an 'easy' baby, a baby that's sweet and loving and even fun. The reality is that the arrival of a new baby is a huge change for the entire family. On a scale of one to ten, a 'normal' baby changes your life by about nine – and a colicky baby changes it by about a thousand.

Don't get trapped into feeling that you have to be there for your baby every minute of every day. A stressed-out, exhausted parent is probably more of a threat to a child's well-being than colic ever could be. Take care of yourself; watch out for signs of depression and sleep deprivation.

When colic threatens to overwhelm you, express a bottle of breastmilk and get away for a while. Give the baby to your partner and go somewhere special, just for you. Remember that colic is only temporary. Your entire family can get through this and move on to the truly wonderful times that lie ahead for all of you.

CHAPTER 10
Special Circumstances

No food can help your baby grow strong and develop intellectually as well as the milk your body produces naturally. That's especially true when your baby faces challenges others don't. Your body will respond to your baby's special needs with special breastmilk. Sometimes, breastfeeding your baby won't be easy, but if you stay with it, the rewards for the entire family will make it all worthwhile.

Premature Infants

These babies are often unable to nurse because of medical interventions and their inability to coordinate a sucking pattern. They are also often fed through a gavage tube that's inserted through the mouth and into the stomach. Human milk is the food of choice for fragile infants. The incredible power of your milk, which is specially developed for your premature infant, will help your baby gain weight, and will also protect him in his already compromised state. Your baby will develop more quickly and be less susceptible to infections when he gets your milk, and you'll feel more connected to him and confident in your abilities as a mother.

What You Can Do

Mothers of premature infants are advised to begin using a breast pump as soon as practical after delivery. Frequent pumping will ensure a good milk supply, regardless of how well your baby can latch or suckle. Try to express milk every two to three hours. Every little bit helps, so don't worry about volume at first – initially, you'll produce just a few drops of colostrum, but that's enough. Colostrum is powerful stuff.

With any baby in a special circumstance, the advice and support of a lactation consultant can make all the difference. At the same time, support groups such as La Leche give you access to other women who've successfully met the same challenges that you and your child face.

Let the hospital staff know that you'll provide your milk for all of your baby's feedings. Leave instructions that your expressed milk should be given to your premature baby with a syringe or a spoon. Finger feeding is another method that sometimes works well.

With the help of the hospital staff, begin breastfeeding a premature infant as soon as possible. These babies are small, so pump before you begin. A taut, full breast is hard to fit into a tiny mouth. Pumping also stimulates your letdown reflex, something a premature infant's weak suck might have trouble accomplishing on its own.

Sometimes positioning a small newborn can be difficult. Because their baby's muscles might be underdeveloped, many women find the football, or clutch, hold useful. The football hold helps because it gives you control and support of your child's head and body.

Premature babies have special needs that only your breastmilk can meet. Breastmilk-fed premature infants have been shown to enjoy better general health than formula-fed babies. When you give birth prematurely, your breasts produce a special milk, called preterm, that's higher in calories, proteins and fats to help your baby grow quickly. This superior food for your infant is something that only you can provide.

Kangaroo Care

If your baby was born prematurely or at low birth weight, kangaroo care is a wonderful alternative to incubators. Allowing mums to provide this uniquely tender care, even to babies who are still on respirators, has had some amazing results. Babies who receive kangaroo care:

· Have more regular heartbeats
· Suffer from less sleep apnoea
· Are more able to regulate their body temperature
· Gain weight more rapidly
· Sleep better
· Are more successful at breastfeeding.

With kangaroo care, the baby is held skin-to-skin on his mother's chest, between her breasts and under her shirt or nightgown. The baby is kept warm, he can hear the heartbeat and breathing he heard in the womb, and he has instant access to the breast. Most health-care providers recommend that periods of kangaroo care should last a short time, such as an hour, to begin with, and slowly increase in duration. In some cases, your first experience might last only a few minutes.

Nurse-midwife Susan Luddington introduced kangaroo care to the United States, from where it spread through the Western world. She had travelled to Bogota, Colombia, and had seen it used in hospitals that lacked isolation cubicles for newborns. Skin-to-skin care was their low-tech solution, and the results are remarkable.

With the exception of breastfeeding, a father is just as capable of providing the benefits of kangaroo care as a mum is. This can be a good opportunity for your partner to bond with your baby – and a good opportunity for you to take a break.

Multiple Births

One of the challenges multiple births often have to overcome is premature birth. Low birth weight and other complications of prematurity make it especially important for twins and triplets to get all the health benefits your milk provides. If your babies are confined to NICU or unable to feed at your breast for other medical reasons, they still benefit from your breastmilk. Follow the advice on premature infants in the section above, and remain confident.

All the regular recommendations given to nursing women go double (or triple) for mothers of multiples: get lots of rest, make sure to drink plenty of water and eat a healthy diet. Feeding more than one baby takes a lot out of you, so you've got to take extra care of yourself. In addition to lots of time, support and supplies, you'll need a feeding strategy – will you nurse them one at a time or together?

One at a Time

If you choose to nurse your infants individually, your partner can keep one entertained while you feed the other. He can sing and cuddle the waiting child or even offer the baby a clean finger to suck on. Once a good nursing routine is established (in about six weeks), your partner can offer one of the babies a bottle of expressed breastmilk – alternate which baby gets the breast first at each feeding, or you might end up with a child who prefers the bottle.

Individual feedings give you a wonderful opportunity to spend quality one-on-one time with each of your precious babies. However, while this is a great approach for bonding, some mothers may feel a bit overwhelmed by the almost constant nursing.

Two Breasts, No Waiting

Most mothers of multiples find that feeding both babies at once is an effective way to streamline the nursing process and make some free time for other activities. Multiples are usually comforted by each other's presence, so they might actually prefer to dine together – after all, they shared some pretty crowded living space for those first nine months!

When both babies nurse at once, they'll probably sleep at the same time, too. Remember, when your babies sleep, you sleep, too. If you're not tired enough to nap, make sure you have a little time to yourself. You've earned it.

Tandem Nursing Supplies

Pillows are the single most important breastfeeding accessory when you're nursing two babies at once. Unless you happen to resemble Shiva, the Indian goddess with eight arms, you won't be able to hold two babies and manipulate two breasts simultaneously.

Pillows raise both babies to the correct height for nursing and keep them safely in position while leaving your hands free. Usually you'll want a pillow on each side of you, and two more pillows to go on your lap. After a while, you'll be able to feed both your babies at once and still have a hand free to hold your glass of water or catch one of your little wiggleworms if he squirms out of position.

Tandem Nursing Positions

The football hold and the crisscross hold are the two most commonly used positions for breastfeeding twins simultaneously. However, any position that works for you is also fine. Some women prefer to lie down and lay one baby over their shoulder and the other in an armpit; experiment until you find a position that you like. Any position you end up using should meet at least the following criteria.

FIGURE 10-1:
Football
(clutch) hold

FIGURE 10-2:
Crisscross
hold

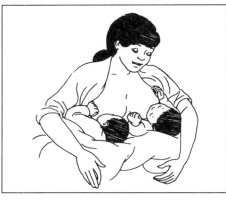
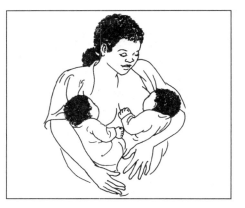

FIGURE 10-3:
Layered hold

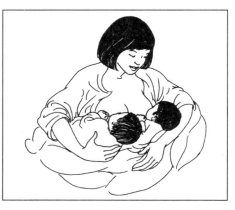

It will take flexibility, patience and practice for all of you to work out which method and position works best for you. Pay extra attention to the babies' position, both to ensure that you're not putting additional strain on your neck and back, and to prevent poor (or sliding) latch from hurting your nipples.

Safety – from falling or suffocation.
Mobility – lets you keep at least one hand free.
Bonding – allows skin-to-skin contact, smell, voice and (ideally) sight.
Positioning – allows proper latch-on and alignment of babies' heads and bodies.

Comfort – for everyone involved.

Longevity – can be maintained for long periods of time.

Triplets

When it's time to breastfeed triplets, you can only feed two at a time. As soon as one finishes, let the third baby nurse. Another option is to give the third infant a bottle of expressed milk while your other two nurse. Put the third infant in his car seat or carrier and rock him until it's his turn. Always rotate feedings so each baby waits in turn.

Milk Supply

The key to building and maintaining an adequate milk supply is frequent feedings at the breast. You can easily produce plenty of milk for twins and even triplets – it's simply a matter of supply and demand. If your babies are frequent, eager nursers, your breasts will increase production and you should then have no problem producing enough milk if you follow a few basic guidelines.

It's best to avoid using a bottle to feed expressed milk to your infants until they've established a strong nursing routine. Bottle feeding can lead to nipple confusion in newborns, as babies suck differently on bottle teats than they do on breasts. A baby who gets used to a bottle might breastfeed less effectively, causing your milk production to decrease. If you have to supplement nursing in the first few weeks of life, use a feeding technique that doesn't involve a teat, such as a spoon or cup.

If you suspect your milk supply is inadequate, evaluate your babies' progress using the information in Chapter 7. The best way to ensure that your babies get what they need is to simply let them nurse often. If frequent nursing doesn't seem to be working, contact your GP or health visitor immediately.

In order to maintain equal milk production in both breasts, alternate sides between babies at a regular interval. You can rotate every feeding, every day or anywhere in between. Whatever schedule you decide on should be easy to remember.

Some women don't alternate sides; they assign a breast to each baby and nurse only him on that breast. The only effect this is likely to have is that one breast might get larger than the other if one baby is a more vigorous feeder.

If your babies can't adequately stimulate your milk production, use a breast pump. This technique is often utilized when a mother is unable to nurse her child directly because of hospitalization or some other necessary separation. If pumping becomes necessary, you should do it at the times your infants would normally nurse. To increase your milk supply, pump more frequently – it's frequency, not duration, that builds a milk supply.

Caesareans

A Caesarean section delivery necessitates some special attention for breastfeeding. As soon as you know you'll be having a Caesarean section, it's important that you remind your doctor of your desire to breastfeed your baby. Let him or her know that you want to breastfeed immediately following birth. Your doctor and the anaesthetist will work with you, providing anaesthesia and follow-up pain medications that are compatible with lactation.

A Caesarean section is major surgery, and your body needs time to recover. Follow your doctor's instructions. Bed rest is often advised even after you return home. Your baby can stay in the room with you, either next to the bed in a crib or beside you in bed. Keep your supplies within arm's reach and rely on your partner or another helper as much as possible. When you feel up to it – and only when you do – get out of bed and walk around. Movement helps you heal. Just take it slowly and carefully, and you'll be all right.

You may find it more comfortable to breastfeed while lying on your side. Lie your baby on a pillow to bring her to the correct height. Babies born via Caesarean section may be drowsy in the early days, due to the anaesthesia, so they may need extra encouragement to feed.

Down's Syndrome

Many babies with Down's syndrome can nurse without too much difficulty, but some do experience some problems with feeding in the early days. Down's babies tend to have less muscle tone, so take special care supporting the baby's head – the football hold allows the most control over your baby's position. Down's babies can also have problems learning to suck, swallow and breathe simultaneously, so it is not uncommon for them to choke and splutter while feeding. These problems often settle down during the first two weeks, however.

If your baby has problems in the early days, you may have more success with expressed breastmilk. If you are feeding your baby from a bottle, there are special teats available for babies who have trouble feeding. Babies with Down's tend to feed slowly, so do not hurry your baby.

Cleft Lip or Cleft Palate

A baby with a cleft lip can usually feed at the breast without much difficulty. If the cleft interferes with his suck, you can cover it with your finger or by pushing a fold of breast tissue into it.

Cleft lips are usually repaired within the first few weeks of life. Some doctors advise against breastfeeding until the lip is healed, but this isn't usually necessary. Many mothers put their babies to breast immediately following surgery – the babies are comforted by nursing, and the mother's milk supply is maintained. If you choose not to nurse straight away, you should pump your breasts to maintain your milk production.

Cleft palates can present more of a challenge, since babies with cleft palates are often unable to keep the breast in their mouths and may have difficulty compressing the milk sinuses beneath the areola. In addition, they tend to get milk into their ears and sinuses through the hole in their palate.

Common solutions include:

· Using the fingers of the hand supporting your breast to hold your baby's head in place. Your palm supports your breast.

- Keeping your baby's head slightly higher than your nipple to prevent milk from flowing into the cleft.
- Changing the angle at which your baby takes the breast, especially by aiming the nipple away from the opening in his palate.
- Using a dental appliance to cover the hole in the palate.

More serious cases might require the use of a special feeding device, such as a soft cup. Your GP or health visitor can help make breastfeeding work for you and your cleft-palate baby.

Tongue Tie

In a tongue-tied baby, the frenulum, the thin line of tissue that connects the tongue to the bottom of the mouth, is short and tight. The baby's tongue can't extend past the bottom teeth or effectively compress the milk sinuses when breastfeeding.

FIGURE 10-4:
Tongue tie

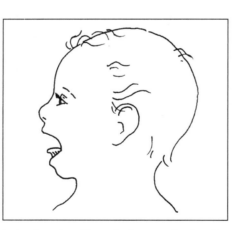

Babies with this condition generally grow out of it, but in the meantime, nursing can be uncomfortable for mum and unsatisfying for baby. If tongue tie interferes with breastfeeding, talk to your doctor.

The clipping of the frenulum is very minor oral surgery. This simple medical procedure takes just minutes and can even be performed by a dentist. Your baby can be back at your breast immediately and nursing will be much improved, but the benefits go beyond breastfeeding – untreated tongue tie can also interfere with speech development.

Relactating and Adoptive Moms

If you've breastfed before but had to stop, it is possible to relactate. Amazingly, it's also possible to induce lactation when you've never given birth or even been pregnant. Inducing lactation lets adoptive mums and their babies enjoy the special advantages of a breastfeeding relationship.

You'll need to pump every two to four hours, day and night, if you plan to induce lactation. Your new baby will nurse that often, so you need to 'tell' your breasts the schedule. A powerful breast pump is your best bet. Some women start to produce milk within three weeks, while others may need six weeks or more. If you're relactating, the rule of thumb states that it will take at least the same amount of time to begin lactating as has passed since you weaned, so if it's been six weeks since you breastfed, it will probably take six weeks to fully relactate. You'll have more success if you enlist the aid of your health visitor or GP.

If you're planning on breastfeeding an adopted baby, remember that most adoptive mums need to supplement their breastmilk with formula. Adoptive breastfeeding is best thought of as a psychological experience, not an exclusively nutritional one. However, there are rare cases where women do manage to produce enough milk for exclusive breastfeeding.

Lactation consultants usually recommend a three-step feeding process for relactating.

1. If possible, breastfeed for a few minutes to encourage the baby to associate the breast with feeding. Provide skin-to-skin contact.
2. Supplement the feeding with a supplemental feeding device that can be used while baby nurses.
3. Pump using a high-quality breast pump.

When the time comes to put your baby to the breast, once again you have to be patient. Many older babies are often a little reluctant to nurse from a breast at first, as they've been bottle fed and may need time to become accustomed to the breast.

Try not to become discouraged if you have little or no visible milk production while pumping. There's something about a real baby, her smell or the feel of her in your arms, that jump-starts lactation like nothing else. Close your eyes while pumping and think about the baby you're going to be holding soon. Creative visualization can affect your whole body.

If your baby is extremely hungry and you're not yet producing much milk, she might be frustrated. Try feeding her a little expressed milk or formula from a spoon or syringe before you breastfeed, or consider using a supplemental feeding device. Put your baby to breast whenever she wants to nurse, but keep it a pleasant experience for both of you. Remember that any human milk is better than none, and the strength of your relationship with your baby is your primary concern.

CHAPTER 11

Nursing on the Go

There's nothing more convenient than breastfeeding when you're on the road. Nature has provided almost everything your baby needs in one convenient package – you! Whether you and your child are going to the super-market or hopping on an international flight, breastfeeding can be a simple, safe and comfortable part of your itinerary.

Nursing in Public

Many women feel comfortable nursing their baby wherever they happen to be. It's every breastfeeding pair's right, and should never be a cause of shame. Still, some women are understandably uncomfortable with the idea of exposing their breasts in public for any reason. We've grown up in a society that promotes the sexuality of breasts over their functionality, but no one should have to feel embarrassed about feeding her child the way nature intended.

There's really not much to see anyway. Many women use a baby blanket or other material to drape over both baby and breast while baby feeds. This can be effective, but it can also draw attention to the whole process, not to mention blocking eye contact with your child. The best way to begin a public nursing session is to simply turn away from view and allow your baby to latch onto the breast. Older nurslings are so adept at the process that you can get them to your breast without much worry about exposing your nipple, even if you don't turn around.

If you're shy at first, your partner can help by acting as a barrier, shielding you from view as baby latches on. A father's support of public nursing can be a real blessing for a shy mother. Not only does a woman need her partner's support in general, but people are much less inclined to look at a breastfeeding pair when Dad's around.

Once your baby has latched onto the breast, her head will conceal it from view, allowing you to nurse comfortably without concern. However, if your baby likes to release the breast every once in a while and look around, be prepared for a little exposure.

Some older babies like to explore their mother's body while they nurse, their busy little hands pulling at clothing and skin alike. If this describes your child, it's a good idea to keep her hands occupied so she doesn't pull up your shirt and expose your other breast. Hold her hands while she nurses, or give her a blanket to cuddle.

Clothing

The right wardrobe is vital for nursing on the go. A two-piece outfit with a top that can be easily pulled up or unbuttoned from the bottom for easy access is best – try an oversized T-shirt or sweatshirt. For women who prefer dresses, some manufacturers offer attractive designs with cleverly concealed vertical openings for quick access. A little extra material, such as pleats or flaps, provides additional cover once baby has latched on.

The choice of material and design is important, too. Cotton prints are the most suitable fabrics for breastfeeding mothers. Cotton breathes, so your baby can be comfortable snuggled against it. Printed designs help to camouflage any wet spots from leaking milk.

Where to Nurse

Many breastfeeding-friendly shops, shopping centres, restaurants and theme parks offer special areas where you can feed your child in a private and comfortable setting. While these areas are often welcome, you're never required to use any special place for breastfeeding – however, many women are a little self-conscious about nursing in public, and, for them, these special areas can be a godsend.

If you're more comfortable nursing privately, here are a few other places to try:

- A corner restaurant booth with your back to the room
- In a car park in your car
- A department store fitting room
- The back pew or child area at church
- The back row at a cinema
- A quiet aisle at the bookstore or library

It is your right to breastfeed wherever you happen to be when your child is hungry. With experience, you'll learn which options provide you with enough privacy and comfort to breastfeed successfully.

Babywearing

If you want real freedom to nurse anywhere, consider babywearing. Slings keep your hands free while holding your baby right where you want her. The extra folds of cloth let you cover both your child and your breast, so you can nurse discreetly as you shop, eat in a restaurant or stand in line at Beanoland or Alton Towers.

Babywearing has other benefits, too: it keeps your little one warm and secure and promotes a healthy emotional attachment; carried babies cry less than other babies and gain weight quicker; parents enjoy a calmer, healthier child and find it easier to care for older siblings when they don't have to use both hands to support a baby. Babywearing is also great exercise for you.

To begin a breastfeeding session using a sling, position your baby on the breast and use one of your hands to keep your little one in place as you walk. You can start moving as soon as your nursling latches on, but try to keep your pace slow and even.

When to Nurse

If you don't like to nurse in public, timing your trips out of the house can be a great help. Since you can't refuse your hungry baby for long, the best strategy is to make sure she's full before you leave home. If you're going to the supermarket, get everything ready and then wait until your baby's next nursing session. The moment she's finished, strap her into the car seat carrier and head out the door. Older children respond well to the same strategy and can even use a dummy or a cup to extend the time between nursing sessions.

If it does become necessary to breastfeed in public, you'll draw much less attention if you begin at the first signs of hunger. If you delay a feeding until your child is crying, everyone will be looking at you as you struggle to get your screaming baby onto the breast. Watch for hunger cues and find a comfortable spot for feeding as soon as your baby lets you know she's ready.

Supplies

Unlike bottle feeding, breastfeeding doesn't tie you down. When you want to go, there's really nothing that you need to take besides your baby, a car seat and maybe a spare nappy or two. You won't need to pack bottles, mix formula or carry as many burping cloths as for a bottle-fed baby.

However, while nature gave you everything you need, there are a few additional items that you might want.

- ❏ Baby sling
- ❏ Comfortable nursing bra
- ❏ Clothing that provides easy, discreet access to your breasts
- ❏ A bottle of water for yourself
- ❏ Nappies
- ❏ Baby wipes
- ❏ Burping cloths
- ❏ Rattle or teething toy (non-chokeable)
- ❏ Extra-large resealable (or recyclable) plastic bags for dirty items
- ❏ Extra outfit for baby (and a T-shirt for you)
- ❏ Dummy for infants older than six weeks
- ❏ Lightweight baby blanket

On long journeys without your baby, you should plan to pack:

- ❏ Manual or battery-operated breast pump
- ❏ Spare batteries and pump parts
- ❏ Storage containers
- ❏ Insulated bag large enough to transport all your expressed milk

Travelling with infants is complicated enough with car seats, buggies and and changing bags; it only gets worse when you add jars of baby food to your load. Breastfeeding makes it possible for you to take advantage of your relative freedom within the first six months.

Travel by Car

Road trips with your child can be a doddle. There's something almost magical about the way a moving vehicle lulls a baby to sleep, and many parents will testify to the calming effect of a little drive. There are even devices on the market that claim to simulate the sensation of a running car when hooked onto a baby's crib.

On long road journeys, the combination of breastfeeding and riding in the car works to your advantage. If you feed your baby before you begin the drive, you can probably expect her to fall asleep in the car and doze contentedly through the first hour or two of travel. When she wakes up, take a break. Pull into a rest area or any convenient car park and feed her. Get out and stretch your legs. Take your baby for a brief stroll, change her nappy and get ready for the next leg of your journey.

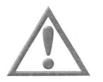

Never remove your child from his car seat for a feeding unless the car is safely parked. All children need to be secured in approved safety restraints whenever the car is on the road. Fretful babies can be calmed with music, toys or even a clean finger to suck on.

On long rides, babies will often sleep more than they would at home. While that makes for a peaceful drive, all that rest can leave your child up later at night than you'd like. It's a good idea to wake your baby at least every three hours for a feeding. You might even want to keep your baby awake as long as possible as you near your destination.

Another alternative used by parents of young children is to travel at night. With your children sleeping peacefully for long stretches of time, you can cover a lot of distance without interruptions. The car is quiet and the traffic is usually light.

Travel by Plane

If you're uncomfortable nursing in public, you might be worried about travelling by plane with your baby. However, the high-backed seats of most commercial airliners give you a fairly private setting for nursing. The only people who can see you are the ones seated in the same row as you, and anyone who walks past. With that in mind, it's usually best to ask for a window seat near the middle of the plane, with your partner or travelling companion seated next to you. The majority of passenger foot travel goes towards the toilets at the front and back of larger aircraft. When you're seated in the middle, passersby will be kept to a minimum, and with your partner blocking the view of the rest of the row of seats, you can feed your baby in privacy.

f(act

Most airlines allow you to bring a car seat carrier onboard with you, even if you haven't paid for your child's seat. As long as the flight isn't fully booked, you can use it. Ask a flight attendant to help you move to a pair of empty seats if the flight is an open one.

If you find yourself in a plane with only one toilet, try to book a seat as far away from it as possible. If all else fails, ask your flight attendant for assistance. He or she will be able to get you a blanket to use as a screen, along with extra pillows. There might even be a more private seat available that you can use.

Ideally, you want your baby to be breastfeeding at takeoff and landing. These are the times when the air pressure in the cabin is changing quickly and can cause ears to pop. Sucking and moving the jaws help to equalize the pressure within your baby's ears by way of the eustachian tubes that connect her ears to her mouth; this is the same relief you get when you chew gum or suck a boiled sweet.

Depending on your travel time to the airport, your check-in time and boarding delays, it might work to your advantage to feed your baby just before leaving the house. Sometimes, however, things just don't work out in your favour, and you'll find yourself with a hungry baby as you wait in the airport terminal. If she seems hungry, nurse her in the terminal – a deserted passenger gate can be a comfortable and private location. Nurse her again at takeoff, as even if she's not hungry, she'll probably suckle for comfort.

Immunization Recommendations

If you're planning to travel abroad, you might need some immunizations depending on your destination. According to current medical guidelines, all immunizations currently given to travellers are compatible with breastfeeding. However, breastfeeding mothers should also be aware that many of the immunities they acquire through immunization will not necessarily protect their nursing children. It's also not safe to give babies those particular injections directly.

Children are immunized according to a well-established schedule that takes into account their physical development. Most authorities recommend that this normal immunization schedule be followed, regardless of your travel destination.

Parents of newborns are advised to seriously consider the risk of disease in certain parts of the world. Infants in the first few months of life are especially vulnerable to infectious diseases.

What can you do to protect your child? Women with infants or toddlers should breastfeed throughout their trip. Breastfeeding enhances a child's immune system, protecting her from a whole host of infections. As an added benefit, breastfed children aren't exposed to potentially impure local water supplies and foods.

Going Solo

If your work includes a long-distance trip or two where you will be unable to take your baby, you'll have to pack a breast pump. Because your milk production is based on supply and demand, you will need to express your milk regularly while you're away from your child. You can pump and dump, pump and donate your milk to a local milk bank (do some research to find one before you travel) or pump and store.

Expressed milk can be stored at room temperature for up to four hours (room temperature must be below 25°C/76°F), for up to 24 hours in a sterile bottle in the refrigerator or frozen for three months. Leave freshly expressed milk to cool in the fridge before adding it to the milk in the freezer. To defrost, hold the container under cold running water then gradually increase the temperature of the water until it reaches room temperature. Do not be tempted to thaw the milk in a microwave, because this can create hot spots in the milk that can burn your baby.

Remember to pack extra batteries for handheld pumps, and to purchase appropriate electrical adaptors if you are travelling abroad. Additional spare parts and collection containers can be hard to find when you're out of the country, so pack those, too.

If your travels include overseas destinations, you will need to express some milk during the flight for comfort. Again, make sure you bring either a battery-operated pump or a manual model; most aircraft don't have electricity available to passengers outside the toilets.

In the event that you find yourself away from home without a pump, hand expression is a viable option. However, you probably won't be able to express enough milk to maintain your supply using hand expression alone. If you plan to continue breastfeeding your baby when you return home, you'll need to remove as much milk as possible. Hand expression is really best utilized as a comfort measure to relieve engorgement; purchase a good pump as soon as possible.

Nursing on the go can be a liberating experience. Anywhere it's appropriate to bottle feed, it's appropriate to breastfeed.

CHAPTER 12

Express Yourself

Madonna did it. So did Kate Winslet, Patsy Palmer, Celine Dion, Cindy Crawford, Sophie Ellis-Bextor, Lisa Kudrow and Mel B. They were all nursing mums who breastfed and expressed milk for their babies. Whether you're returning to work, relieving engorgement or pumping milk so you can have a night out, at some point all nursing mothers need to learn the art of expression.

Pump It Up!

A breast pump is not as effective in removing milk from your breasts as your baby is, so it's important to establish a consistent routine to maintain your supply. The more frequently you pump, the stronger your supply will be, just as frequent nursing works with your baby.

A New Routine

Begin to express your milk about two weeks before returning to work. This will help increase your production and get you into a pumping routine. You'll want to express about the same time as your baby would naturally nurse each day, or about every two to three hours in any 24-hour period.

Begin pumping for 15 minutes using a double pump, or 30 minutes using a single pump (15 minutes on each side).

How can you tell if you are expressing a 'normal' amount of milk?
Breasts develop their own general flow pattern. They start dripping, then squirt, then drip, then slow to stop. Continue to pump until the milk stops flowing or dripping.

You might notice that not much milk is expressed the first few times you try. It takes time for your body to get used to this artificial suction device, and it also takes time for your milk to let down. Eventually you'll notice steady streams and bona-fide long-distance sprays from your nipples, but don't worry about that now – any milk you express is important for your baby's growth. After about a week, you should be able to pump up to 750ml (25fl oz) or more per day.

When Should I Pump?

Your prolactin levels fluctuate throughout the day; they're lowest in the evening and highest in the morning. If you express your milk in the morning, you will have greater volume. Pump before you wake your baby.

You can still nurse her because your breasts are never really empty. Pump again one and a half to two hours later.

Milk flows best when you're relaxed. If you have difficulty with letdown when you pump, nurse your baby on one breast while pumping the other. Once your baby engages your milk ejection reflex, your milk will flow more freely.

Manual Expression

Sometimes, particularly if you are engorged, your baby might have a difficult time finding enough nipple to take into her mouth. You might need to express some milk manually to relieve the fullness in your breasts and provide some elasticity to your nipple and areola.

Manual expression is the least expensive kind of 'pumping'. It can be easy with practice, but it can be difficult to learn, and if done incorrectly, it can cause bruising, tissue damage or chafed skin. Ask your health-care provider to demonstrate the correct technique, since seeing it in action is different from reading about it in a book. Practise manual expression even if you don't intend to make it a daily routine – at some point you might need to express your milk without the use of a pump.

FIGURE 12-1:
Breast
massage

FIGURE 12-2:
Manual
expression

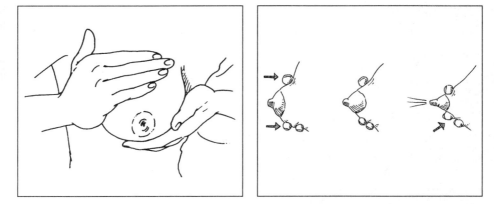

Eventually you can try the two-handed, doubled-breasted method while sitting at a table and expressing milk into a large pan or bowl. If you don't intend to store your milk for later, you can also express your milk in a warm shower.

HOW TO EXPRESS MANUALLY

1. Wash your hands and get a clean collection container. A wide-mouth cup strategically placed in front of the nipple will catch your milk as it squirts. Some mothers place a funnel inside a baby bottle to collect their milk.

2. Gently massage your breasts. Use small circular motions as if you're conducting a breast self-examination, or do whatever feels comfortable. Start on the outside of the breast and move towards the areola; bend over at the waist and let gravity assist you. The key is to relax and allow letdown to occur. Warm flannels applied to the breast will also help.

3. Place your thumb and first two fingers about 25mm (1in) behind the nipple or on the edge of the areola in a twelve o'clock and six o'clock position. Your fingers will resemble the letter C.

4. Lift your breast and push it back towards your ribcage.

5. Press down towards the nipple in a gently rolling motion to compress milk out of the sinuses, the way your baby does when she nurses. Don't squeeze the nipple, just the sinuses under the areola. Release your hold and do this again.

6. When milk begins to flow, rotate your hand position around the breast (i.e. at eleven and five o'clock) and continue until the sinuses are empty. Work all sides of the breast until milk no longer flows or drips.

7. Rub excess milk onto your nipple and areola.

Breast Pump Selection

If you intend to express your milk on a regular basis, you'll want to choose a breast pump that meets your individual needs; the criteria vary from person to person, and even over time for the individual. Keep your ultimate goal (whatever it may be) in mind while you shop, and consult your doctor or health visitor.

- How often will you use a pump: daily, weekly, or as needed? Are you returning to work or just planning to express an occasional bottle for a night out?

- What can you afford? Is this an investment that you intend to use again with other babies, or would it be more economical for you to hire?
- Will you be transporting your breast pump to work? Will you need a cooler or carrying case to carry milk home again?
- Will you be expressing in your car?
- What are your power sources?
- How much time do you have to express your milk?
- What kinds of accessories will you need?

When choosing a pump, select the one that most closely imitates your baby's suckling pattern. Pumps that offer the most cycling per minute are the best – look for ones that offer 34–50 cycles per minute, as this timing is most like your baby's nursing pattern. You'll also want a pump with adjustable suction rates.

Where can I find more information about hiring breast pumps?
The companies listed below are leaders in hiring breast pumps, and their pumps are supplied to most hospitals and maternal/child health organizations.

When selecting a breast pump, you really do get what you pay for. Better pumps will cost more, but they are able to express more milk in a shorter period of time, are more comfortable to use and are less likely to cause tissue damage.

Contact your health visitor or a breastfeeding counsellor about the different pumps available. They'll share the pros and cons of each model with you and can give you additional information about where to purchase or hire a good-quality pump.

NCT Breastfeeding   0870 444 8708
Breastfeeding Network Supporters   0870 900 8787
La Leche League   020 7242 127

Ameda Egnell Ltd	01823 336362
Medela	01538 399541
The Maternity Alliance	020 7588 8583

Types of Breast Pumps

It's important to choose a reputable brand, whose manufacturers have years of experience and a solid history behind their products. A breast pump is an important tool, not a toy – you wouldn't go to a seafood restaurant if you wanted to eat steak, so don't buy a breast pump from a company that specializes in something else.

Reading about breast pumps in consumer product safety reports is a useful way to compare products based on durability, repair frequency, cost and any other criteria that are important to you. It's also the place to find out about safety notes and recalls.

Breast pumps are usually quite product-specific – you may have to use bottles and bags from the same range – so check this before purchasing.

Bicycle Horn Pump

Shaped like a bicycle horn, these pumps are the least expensive, but also the least effective. You create suction by squeezing and releasing the bulb, and milk is collected into the bulb or a depression in the bottom of the horn. However, because the bulbs can't always be disassembled and cleaned, they can become contaminated with bacterial growth. In addition, bicycle horn pumps can cause breast tissue damage. Unless you are pumping and dumping, these are to be avoided.

Hand- or Foot-Operated Pumps

There are several hand pumps on the market, and making a decision about the right one is a difficult task. Most hand pumps offer cylinder-style action or handgrip operation. With cylinder pumps you pull on a piston or plunger to create suction. The flange (a funnel-like contraption) is centred over your nipple and you push the plunger in, then pull it out to draw milk from the breast sinuses.

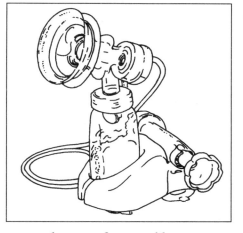

FIGURE 12-3:
One type
of manual
breast pump

Handgrip pumps work in much the same way, providing suction through the squeeze of a bar. These types offer convenient one-handed operation.

Foot-pedal pumps are, as the name implies, manual pumps worked with your feet – a hose runs from the pedal to the flange. Foot-pedal pumps offer double pumping, which is the most effective method of expression.

Each type of manual breast pump is effective and offers good exercise, but might wear you out. These pumps are best for occasional use only.

Handheld Battery-Operated Pumps

Battery-operated pumps use a small motor to produce suction. Some older pumps require you to manually release the suction, while newer models offer automatic or button suction-release. The motor creates a vacuum on your nipple/areola, and you break suction to create the pseudo-nursing effect. Some pumps offer an automatic release that has a cycle of around four to eight times per minute.

Although handheld battery-operated pumps are inexpensive, they are not very efficient and can cause tissue damage. They're generally slower to create and release suction, so their action doesn't mimic your baby's suckling; in fact, they're often responsible for a diminished milk supply. Many of these pumps are poorly constructed and seem to break just before their three-month warranty expires, and in addition, they can be noisy and require frequent battery replacement. They are best used for occasional pumping only.

Portable Electric Pumps

These pumps are durable and easy to transport, but often don't offer the optimum number of suction-release cycles. As with many handheld battery-operated machines, some electric pumps depend on the user to break suction. Portable electric pumps often come with accessory packages that offer cigarette lighter adaptors for use in your car. These pumps are more effective if you have an abundant milk supply, and they also have adjustable suction rates.

Hospital-Grade Pumps

These are simply the best and most efficient pumps around. Although they can be expensive to purchase, most hospitals offer hiring options for women who intend to pump frequently. Hospital-grade pumps come in several sizes and weights, some as light as 1.8kg (4lb), while others can weigh up to 8.9kg (20lb). The lightweight pumps are easily transported and come with adaptors for use in a car.

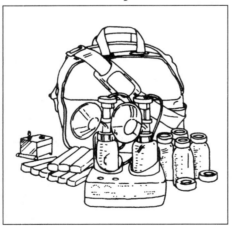

FIGURE 12-4: Hospital-grade pump

Look for a pump that provides an automatic suction-release cycle that mimics your baby's suck. Most cycle around 48–60 times per minute. These pumps offer double pumping, are great for establishing a strong milk supply, and are perfect for the working mother or for use when you have a child in hospital.

Sometimes the costs of hiring hospital-grade pumps can be covered by medical insurance, particularly if your baby is premature or has a medical condition – the author's doctor wrote a letter to the insurance company about the benefits of breastfeeding a low-birth-weight infant, and they covered all pump expenses for six months. Hospital-grade pumps are the most effective as well as cost-efficient, if you use them on a daily basis – the fees can be calculated daily, weekly or monthly.

Pump Process (20–30 Minutes)

1. Wash your hands with soap and water.
2. Wash all breast pump equipment and assemble it according to the manufacturer's directions.
3. Find a comfortable location to express, just as you would to nurse your baby.
4. Gently massage your breasts or apply a warm flannel.
5. Centre the nipple in the plastic flange. If you are using an electric or battery-operated pump, turn it to the lowest/slowest setting first and increase the speed to match your baby's suck. If you are using a cylinder pump, pull the piston away from your breast, push it back in and pull it out again. Try to mimic one suck per second.

 Watch how your nipple enters and exits the flange – if your nipple is squashed, you might need a larger flange neck, as nipples should not rub or touch the sides. Contact the outlet you purchased your kit from to see about their exchange policy.

6a. Pump the first breast for about seven minutes. (If you are using a double pump, note that you'll follow the pump–massage–pump procedure without switching breasts.)
6b. Switch sides and pump the second breast for seven minutes.
7. Massage your breasts a second time.
8. Return to the first breast for five to seven minutes or until milk no longer flows, followed by the second breast for the same amount of time.
   Note: You might have to exchange containers midway through your expression session if your collection bottle becomes full.
9. When milk stops dripping, release suction at the breast as you would with your infant.
10. When you're finished, rub any excess milk onto your nipples and areola.
11. Pour the milk into a clean container for storage, or, if a lid is provided with your pump, screw it on tightly.

12. Label your milk with the date and the amount, and immediately refrigerate what you don't plan to use within eight to ten hours.
13. Detach the pump and disassemble any washable components. Clean everything according to the instructions in hot, soapy water. Air dry the components on a paper towel or a clean tea towel.

Storing Milk

After you've expressed your breastmilk, you will need to store it if it's not immediately given to your baby. Human milk can be stored at room temperature, refrigerated or frozen; each requires different handling and storage procedures. Temperature is the single most important factor in determining the length of time it's safe to store your milk. The guidelines given here are for a full-term, healthy baby. Consult your health visitor if you have any concerns.

STORAGE TIME GUIDELINES	
Room temperature	4 hours below 25°C (76°F)
Refrigerator (4°C/40°F or colder)	24 hours
Freezer inside a refrigerator	2 weeks
Fridge-freezer with separate doors	3 months
Deep freeze (–20°C/–40°F, no defrost cycle)	6–12 months

Defrosted or thawed milk can be stored for up to 24 hours in the refrigerator. If you don't have a refrigerator at your workplace, you can refrigerate milk in an insulated cooler with ice packs until you get home or to where your baby is being looked after.

Store your cooled or frozen milk in the back of your refrigerator. It's cooler there, and your milk will be less affected by temperature changes from frequent opening and closing of the door.

Studies have found that the antibacterial properties of breastmilk actually protect it from bacterial growth while it's stored in a bottle. That's why human milk can be stored at room temperature for up to four hours. However, if you don't intend to use your milk for some time, it's best refrigerated. Discard any unused portion left in the bottle after your baby has eaten. It's hard to watch that liquid gold go down the drain, but bacteria from your baby's mouth make it unsafe for future feedings.

If you are planning to freeze milk, do so within 24 hours of pumping and chill it in the fridge first.

Critically ill infants require different breastmilk handling and storage techniques to full-term, healthy infants. The hospital staff will work closely with you on expression and storage.

Plastic versus Glass Debate

Every couple of years, breastfeeding educators learn about new studies that change the recommended practice for storing human milk. A few years ago, plastic was the container of choice; then there was a concern about chemicals in plastic that might leach into milk. As a result, glass was recommended. Soon afterwards, studies indicated that lycocytes, or living cells, clung to the sides of glass bottles. This made researchers question whether infants were actually receiving all of the benefits of breastmilk. Today, new plastics have been developed in response to chemical leakage concerns, and the recommendation is back to plastic.

Many women freeze breastmilk in both metal and hard plastic ice cube trays; once frozen, the cubes are removed and stored in freezer bags. Current research indicates no harm or benefit with this practice.

Plastic – If you're freezing breastmilk in plastic bottles or liner bags, leave at least 25mm (1in) at the top – as liquids freeze, they expand. Mark the date and amount on the outside of the bottle or bag using wax pencils or masking tape, and add your baby's name if the bottle will be used at a day care centre. If you're freezing breastmilk in a bottle liner, double-bag your milk to decrease the chances of seam leakage. If you have an extra bottle handy, freeze milk with bags still in the bottle to preserve their shape. Bottle liners that are intended for the long-term storage of human milk are the best.

Freeze milk in amounts of 60–125ml (2–4fl oz). This way, it will thaw more quickly and less will go to waste. When baby consistently takes 250ml (8fl oz) at a single feeding, you can safely freeze your milk in larger amounts, but larger amounts take longer to thaw.

Glass – Because milk expands when frozen, be careful to leave adequate space available in the bottle for this process. Glass bottles can break if you fill them all the way to the top. Again, freeze in smaller amounts.

Ice cube trays – Simply pour liquid into a metal tray and seal the whole thing inside a large freezer bag, or cover it tightly with clingfilm or aluminium foil. Pop out the cubes as needed. If the cubes are too large to fit into the mouth of the bottle, thaw them inside the refrigerator in another container and transfer the milk to a bottle when it's ready.

Sterilizing containers

All bottles and containers that come into contact with your milk should be scrupulously clean, and for young babies they should be sterilized as well, in order to kill any bacteria. The bottle and teat should be rinsed and washed using a bottle brush to remove any milk deposits. You should also check that the hole in the teat is not blocked, then rinse again. There are different sterilizing methods:

Boiling – You can boil all the equipment in a pan for 10 minutes – make sure everything is completely submerged.

Tablets or liquid – Add sterilizing fluid or tablets to a pan of water and leave for 30 minutes (again, be sure to cover all the equipment).

Steam – An electrical machine will sterilize all your equipment in about 10 minutes

Microwave unit – This is the fastest system, taking about five minutes. Check that all your equipment is safe for use in the microwave.

Thawing Frozen Breastmilk

The recommendation for thawing breastmilk is to let it stand in the refrigerator overnight. Milk will thaw slowly and consistently over a 12-hour period, and faster if frozen in smaller amounts.

Do not refreeze thawed milk or reheat heated milk. Throw away any milk remaining in your baby's bottle, and always use the oldest milk first.

Another common method of thawing milk is to run bottled milk under a warm running tap.

Breastmilk separates into milk and fat (cream). The fat floats to the top. Once your breastmilk is thawed, gently shake or swirl the bottle to mix it all up again. Thawed milk sometimes smells 'soapy', but that doesn't mean it's sour or has gone bad; it usually happens in response to defrosting the fat in the milk.

Heating Fresh Milk

Your breastmilk is the perfect temperature for your baby. Even when it's been stored at room temperature, fresh milk doesn't need to be heated. Boiling causes the milk to lose its precious immunity-enhancing properties, and even a slight warm-up in the microwave can hurt the milk and possibly harm your baby, as microwave heat is uneven and causes hot spots in a bottle that will scald her mouth. If you decide to refrigerate your milk, you can heat it by holding the bottle under warm tap water or letting it stand in a bowl or pan of warm water.

It's best to use your breastmilk in the first few days after you've expressed it. Breastmilk is filled with living cells and delicate ingredients that are meant for your child immediately and loses many of its disease-fighting properties with freezing or boiling, and over a period of time. Although it's still the most perfect nutrition for your child, the near-magical immunity properties of your milk are important, too.

Pump Up the Volume!

Your milk supply will decrease the first week you return to work. If that return happens at six weeks post partum, your baby also hits a growth spurt at this time. Remember to express milk frequently on a regular schedule to keep up with your baby's demands. Nurse as soon as you greet your infant, even if it's in your child-care provider's home. Your milk supply will catch up within a few days.

What about Dads?

Get Dad to set up the pump and keep you supplied with warm flannels. If you prefer to pump in privacy, make it your partner's special time with your new baby. Dad can help out by making your pumping experience as relaxing as possible. Anything that helps you relax also helps you to let down your milk – a good foot-rub while you pump can be wonderful, as can a shoulder massage. If he can control himself, teach him the fine art of breast massage.

If you've begun to offer your baby an occasional bottle of expressed milk, this is the perfect time for your partner to participate in the feeding of your baby. A bottle of expressed milk in the refrigerator means that anyone can handle those midnight feedings. Let the games begin...

CHAPTER 13

Bottle Feeding Your Baby

f you've been nursing your baby at all, you've given your baby a loving, healthy start. If you're going to bottle feed now, you need to make a few informed decisions. Are you going to continue with breastmilk or switch to formula, or use both? If you choose to add formula to your routine, how does that work? And then there are bottles and nipples to consider.

Bottles, Teats and Other Supplies

Whether you are incorporating formula into your routine or need bottles for expressed milk, your considerations will be the same: comfort and safety for your child, and simplicity for you. Remember that your child is used to your breast, so it's important to find a product to which he can adjust easily.

Bottles

Bottles come in two sizes: 120ml (4fl oz) and 225ml (7fl oz); the smaller size is suitable for newborns and the larger for older babies. Basic bottles are relatively inexpensive, which is fortunate, as you will need several, even if you are just expressing milk. Remember that cleaning, sterilizing and drying your bottles takes time, and you don't want to have to hunt around for a clean one. Additionally you are probably planning to store some expressed milk in bottles, so buy plenty (about six is usually sufficient).

If your baby has been breastfed exclusively for at least 12 months, you can skip this section. Babies that age don't need a bottle and should be ready to go straight to a cup or straw. If you introduced the cup at six months, she's probably an old pro by now. It's easier to wean a baby just once!

Disposable bottles – These ready-sterilized bottles come with a teat and lid, and are suitable for babies from three months old. You simply add the milk then throw away the whole bottle. These are brilliant if you are travelling, but they do work out expensive and do nothing to help the environment.

Anti-colic bottles – As any parent of a baby with colic will tell you, anything that can help is a boon. Many manufacturers have tried to design bottles that reduce the amount of air your baby ingests at a feed – which is thought to be a cause of colic. These vary from bottles that allow air to escape through vents to collapsible bottles. If your baby needs a lot of burping after a bottle feed, you may find these helpful.

Sterilizer bottles – These do not need any other sterilizing equipment than a microwave, so they are very convenient. However, they are also expensive, and are no good at all if you are visiting someone who doesn't have a microwave.

Teats

These can be made from latex or silicone. Silicone is a little less flexible than traditional latex, but is more hard-wearing, and it has no taste of its own. Silicone is also transparent, which means you can see the milk entering the teat. Teats are also available with different flow rates, and generally the slower speeds are better for younger babies.

In addition to standard-shaped teats, you can also buy 'natural' varieties that aim to mimic the shape of the mother's nipple more closely; as with most things 'baby', it is a question of finding what suits you both. Anti-colic teats, like their companion bottles, aim to reduce the amount of air a baby swallows at each feed. Be aware that boiling makes teats deteriorate more quickly than other sterilizing methods.

Make it a habit to check teats for wear and deterioration at every cleaning. Grasp the teat between your thumb and forefinger. Hold the base with your other hand and pull. The teat should snap back firmly. Immediately replace any torn, sticky, swollen or cracked bottle teats.

Dummies

All babies need to suck – even if she isn't hungry, sucking can calm and comfort a fretful baby. Breastfeeding mums are advised against the use of dummies until a solid nursing routine is established, but bottle-fed babies can use them immediately. Try to stick with the same teat design as your baby's bottle.

Dummies are made in one of two ways. One-piece construction means that the entire dummy is moulded at once from the same material. Composite construction means that the teat is attached to separately moulded parts made from different materials. The one-piece style is the safest – it may be a little harder to find, but the extra peace of mind is worth the effort.

DUMMY SAFETY CHECKLIST:
❑ One-piece construction
❑ No attached cord or strings, clips or decorations
❑ Air holes in the shield
❑ Large and firm enough that it cannot bend or fit into baby's mouth

In the USA, the Consumer Products Safety Commission lists dummy recalls on its website going back to 1984. Of the 21 recalls, at least 17 were for composite dummies, and the most common problem was small parts that presented a choking hazard. Just like bottle teats, pacifier teats wear out and become unsafe. Check them after every washing.

Keeping It Clean

All bottles, teats and any other equipment that comes into direct contact with your milk should be washed in warm soapy water using a brush to remove milk residues — then rinsed (or put through the dishwasher). You then need to sterilize the equipment in one of the following ways:

Boiling – Put the equipment in a pan and cover with water, then boil for 10 minutes, making sure the equipment is completely submerged. This is an inexpensive method, but teats do degrade more quickly than with other methods. It may also be awkward to have boiling pans on the stove a lot – especially if you have mobile children.

Cold water sterilizing – This comes in the form of tablets or a liquid that you add to a pan of cold water and leave for about half an hour. This is an inexpensive but time-consuming method, although you can sterilize equipment practically anywhere.

Steam sterilizing – Electric sterilizers hold up to six bottles at a time and work in about 10 minutes. Unopened bottles stay sterile for about three hours. The unit itself is relatively expensive, but it is a one-off cost and this is a very convenient method.

Microwave steam sterilizing – This uses relatively inexpensive containers that fit inside the microwave and use water to create steam. Always check that your equipment is microwaveable. Of course, if you are visiting someone with no microwave you will have to make alternative arrangements.

As you would with any tinned food, wipe the top of the formula tin with a clean cloth before opening. You can be confident that the contents of the tin are clean and safe, but you don't know what's been on the outside.

Always use cooled, boiled fresh water to make up a formula feed.

Formula

Pre-manufactured infant formula is a recent invention. Chemist and merchant Henri Nestlé claimed to produce the first commercially available artificial infant food back in 1867, and the Nestlé Company is still producing infant food today.

Choosing a Formula

Before you feed your newborn anything besides breastmilk, talk to your doctor. There are many different types and brands of infant formula.

Cow's Milk-Based Formula

This is the most widespread of formulas, and is standard fare for most formula-fed babies from birth to their first birthday. Vitamins, minerals, fats and sugars are mixed together in a base of cow's milk proteins. If your baby is normal birth weight and healthy, and if you have no reason to suspect food allergies, a regular formula based on modified cows' milk is usually the right choice.

Many companies are now marketing two types of formula – described as something like 'first stage' and 'hungrier baby'. These have different curds and whey ratios, with the 'hungry' formula taking longer to digest. First-stage milk is suitable up to the age of one year, and switching milk can cause constipation. If your baby does not seem happy with your choice of formula, talk to your health visitor about changing brands or looking for an alternative. Although most baby milk is derived from cow's milk, the BMA advises that babies under one year old should not be given cow's milk in its natural form, only specially designed infant formula.

Follow-Up Formulas

After your baby celebrates her first birthday, she's ready to move beyond formula. Along with all the wonderful new foods your baby's been trying since she was six months old, your baby can now drink milk – plain, ordinary pasteurized whole milk. Follow-up formulas are marketed to parents who are worried about their baby's nutrition – some follow-ups are even marketed to parents of children as young as four months – but there is no real reason to switch from a regular formula at such a young age. If your little one is getting proper nutrition in her diet after her first birthday, follow-up formulas are no more than an unnecessary expense.

Powdered, Concentrated or Ready-to-Feed?

For economy, availability and shelf life, choose powdered formula mix. Powdered is the old, reliable form of infant formula. It's great for around the house, every shop seems to carry it, and the price is right. Of course, the difference in cost is only a few pence less per feeding, but over the course of a month, that can add up to enough cash for, oh, maybe... a baby-sitter? On the down side, formula powder is a little bit messy and preparation is the most complicated (but still pretty simple).

Concentrated liquid is a nice middle ground between the indulgence of ready-to-feed and the savings of powder. Concentrated is nearly as available as powder, and mixing is simple; the cost is right between the other two types of formula, too. Concentrated liquid, however, doesn't work well out of the house, as opened tins need to be refrigerated immediately, and you've got to have safe water for mixing.

Ready-to-feed is the Rolls Royce of formulas. You can buy it in large containers or even individual serving bottles with disposable teats. Sound expensive? It is. The disposable teats seem a little wasteful, too, but don't try to reuse them, as this isn't safe – they are not made for multiple uses. Ready-to-feed formula is unmatched among formulas for travelling convenience: pack a number of single-serving bottles in the changing bag and you're ready for anything.

Feeding with a Bottle

First, get yourself comfortable. Find a place where you can easily support the baby for a length of time without straining yourself. A comfortable chair is a good choice.

Second, tilt the bottle so that the teat fills with formula, otherwise your baby will swallow excessive amounts of air during feeding. More air equals more spit-up.

Third, tilt your baby so that her head is higher than her stomach. Never feed your baby when she is lying down – she can get ear infections, as the Eustachian tubes connect your baby's mouth and inner ear and when she drinks lying back, fluids run into her inner ear and stay there. Any food warmed to body temperature is like a fertility clinic for bacteria. Sitting up or reclining slightly are the correct positions for feeding.

When your baby's first tooth arrives, it's time to begin practising a good dental routine. Buy a soft, child-sized toothbrush or use a wet cloth; you don't need toothpaste at this age. Make a game of cleaning that precious little tooth. Remember, the goal is to take care of the teeth while getting your child into the habit of good dental hygiene.

Fourth, cuddle your baby and hold her as if you were breastfeeding. This is especially true for newborns – a newborn's eyes can't focus well beyond about 30cm (12in) or so, which just happens to be the distance between your eyes and hers when she is breastfeeding. Your baby wants to see you; she wants to interact with you and get to know you. Cuddle your baby while she eats. Coo to her. Sing to her. Take off your shirt and go skin to skin. These activities bring security and comfort to your baby, and help you to bond. Sometimes it might seem as if you've been feeding her forever, but you'll look back on those early feedings fondly when your little baby isn't so little any more.

As your baby becomes able to grasp the bottle and take control, let her. Her coordination might be lacking at first. Sometimes babies frustrate themselves by knocking the bottle out of their own mouths. At those times, hold the bottle but let her grasp and tug it around. Before long, she'll be an old hand.

Dad's Turn

Dads and older siblings have a wonderful opportunity to hold and cuddle their babies during bottle feeding. Take turns with the baby, or feed in shifts. You're a family now; make raising your baby a family affair – if you can all be involved, your baby will thrive. Whether you're using formula or breastmilk, your bottle-feeding experience can be very satisfying.

CHAPTER 14

Nutrition for Mum

Breastfeeding mums have nutritional needs above and beyond those of other women. Your milk quality won't usually suffer from poor eating habits, but your own health might. Your body will provide your baby with all the nutrients she needs, even if it means taking them from itself. Many women don't eat a well-balanced diet, so their bodies rob themselves of important nutrients in order to supply their growing infant's needs.

A Healthy Example

When your toddler sees you enjoying good food, she's more likely to enjoy it herself. If you don't like a particular vegetable, she'll pick up on that, too. Getting your child started with a healthy lifestyle is the loving thing to do, and it can be as simple as having healthy food around the house instead of crisps and sweets.

Fathers can help, too – it's hard to maintain healthy eating habits if your partner isn't following the game plan. Dads should try to stick with a healthy menu around their partners and children whenever possible. It's all too easy to let either parent's bad habit become the family's bad habit. An occasional treat is fine, but if you feel the need to indulge in junk food, practise moderation.

A Word about Water

During lactation, your body uses tremendous amounts of water. While mild dehydration on your part won't affect your milk production in any significant way, it will cause problems for your own overall health. Irritability and a loss of energy and focus are just a couple of common symptoms of dehydration.

Moments after sitting down to breastfeed, you'll begin to feel thirsty; almost every woman does. Get in the habit of taking a glass of water with you every time you nurse. When your baby takes the fluid out, you put it straight back in.

Water is the recommended beverage; juice and soft drinks are too sugary and don't replace your body's fluids as well as water does. A glass or two of fruit juice per day is a healthy addition to your diet, but drinking juice instead of water can lead to unwanted weight gain.

Don't wait until you're thirsty to have a glass of water. Thirst is a late indicator of dehydration. Usually by the time you feel thirsty, your body is already too dry. If your urine is consistently dark, your mouth is dry and you suffer from constipation, you're probably dehydrated. Stay ahead of dehydration by drinking eight to ten glasses of water every day, but don't overdo it: extra water won't increase your milk production.

Food Pyramid

A useful quick reference guide to healthy eating is the Food Pyramid that you may have learned about back in primary school – it's a handy way to put together a healthy daily menu. The pyramid is built from six food groups.

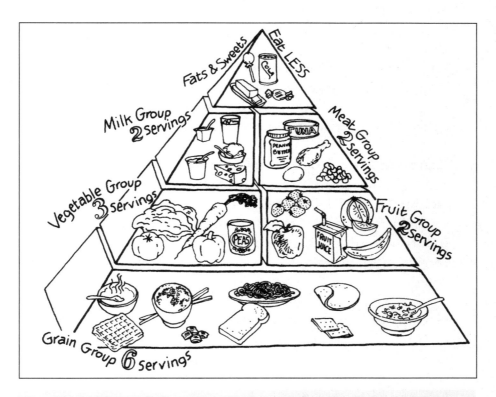

Figure 14-1: Food Pyramid. The Department of Health does ongoing research on nutrition and provides the public with tools to ensure healthy eating habits. Use the Food Pyramid as a guide for yourself, and talk to your GP or health visitor about a similar guide for your child.

Group 1: Bread, Cereal, Rice and Pasta

The grains group is the base of the Food Pyramid, and foods from this group should make up the majority of your daily diet. Six to eleven servings per day are recommended for breastfeeding women. A serving from this group would be a single slice of bread, 30g (1oz) of ready-to-eat cereal, or 90g (3oz) of rice, pasta or cooked cereal.

Group 2: Vegetables

The vegetable group is a rich source of nutrients but is often neglected in many Western diets. Eating the recommended five servings of vegetables per day is a good start. A serving roughly equals 60g (2oz) of raw, leafy vegetables; 30g (1oz) of cooked or chopped raw vegetables; or a glass of vegetable juice.

Group 3: Fruit

Fruits are delicious and nutritious. Just two to four servings per day will keep you in good shape and give your body the natural sugars it craves. A medium-sized whole fruit; 30g (1oz) of chopped, cooked or tinned fruit; or a glass of fruit juice each count as one serving.

Group 4: Milk, Yogurt and Cheese

The dairy group is a great source of calcium and is often fortified with vitamin D. Four daily servings are recommended for women who nurse their babies: 250ml (8fl oz) of milk or yogurt, 185g (6oz) of natural cheese, or 220g (7oz) of processed cheese count as a single serving. It's not necessary to drink lots of extra milk when lactating – you don't need milk in your diet to make milk in your breasts.

Group 5: Meat, Poultry, Fish, Eggs, Nuts and Dried Beans

Incorporate three daily servings from this group, which helps provide essential fats, proteins, vitamins and minerals in a relatively small package. Consider a serving to consist of 60–90g (2–3oz) of cooked lean meat, two eggs, four tablespoons of peanut butter or 150g (5oz) of nuts.

Group 6: Fats, Oils and Sweets

There is no recommended daily intake of foods from group six. Use fats, oils and sweets sparingly. Fats and sugars are important to your health, but most Westerners consume too much of them. All the necessary fat and sugar you need is present in the foods from the other five Food Guide groups in healthier amounts and in combination with other nutrients.

While reviewing 'Nutrition Facts' on food packaging, be aware that the suggested serving sizes listed reflect the amount of food that the producer considers to be one serving. The serving size recommended by the Food Guide Pyramid is based on the amount of the food necessary for your nutritional needs.

Vitamin and Mineral Supplements

The best way to fulfill all your nutritional requirements is by eating a varied diet from the lower five groups of the Food Pyramid. Whole foods are complex powerhouses of good things for your body. A vitamin C pill might provide all your required vitamin C, but an orange provides the same benefit as a pill along with fibre, carotene, calcium, simple sugars and more. Many of the components of whole foods might help us in ways that haven't been discovered yet; we just don't know all there is to know about nutrition. Without a complete knowledge of our nutritional needs, we can't presume to fill those needs with an artificial supplement.

Large doses of otherwise good nutrients can cause health problems: excessive vitamin D can cause symptoms ranging from nausea to kidney failure, while too much vitamin A can lead to headaches, hair loss and liver damage. Avoid taking supplements that contain more than the recommended daily allowance (RDA) of any nutrient.

Another reason why whole foods are superior to supplements is the availability of the nutrients to your body. It's not enough for a pill to contain 100 per cent of your daily vitamin and mineral needs if those nutrients are provided in a form your body can't easily use. The availability of nutrients is sometimes strongly affected by the presence of other nutrients. A multivitamin and mineral pill contains ingredients that get in each other's way – for instance, high doses of iron will interfere with your body's ability to absorb zinc and copper.

This is not to say that you absolutely shouldn't take a daily supplement, but a pill is not a cure for poor eating habits. Think of vitamin and mineral pills as a way to increase your chances of getting all the nutrients you need. Your prenatal supplement is a good source of nutrients that might help to fill in the blanks on your body's nutritional checklist. Avoid taking any additional supplements without the approval of your health-care provider.

Breastmilk and Your Diet

When you eat a rich, varied diet, your baby enjoys a variety of milk flavours. Today, it's a creamy garlic sauce courtesy of last night's Italian dinner. Tomorrow, who knows? Your baby will get her first exposure to the foods you like through the flavour of your milk.

Foods to Avoid

Most women can eat anything they want while breastfeeding, without any problems. However, there are some foods that have a bad reputation among nursing mothers. These foods can pass into your breastmilk and change its flavour or cause allergic reactions in your baby. Symptoms vary, but usually involve fretfulness, an unwillingness to feed, rash, diarrhoea or vomiting. Often a baby who suddenly refuses to nurse is responding to the flavour of your milk. If your baby displays any of these symptoms, examine your diet and check it against this list of the usual suspects.

- Caffeine
- Chocolate
- Citrus fruits
- Dairy products
- Foods that cause wind
- Nuts (especially peanuts)
- Spicy foods

Eliminating these foods from your diet might help. However, the change in your baby will not be immediate. To find the offending food, try cutting out one of the possible culprits from your diet for a week or two. If your baby's symptoms persist, try eliminating the next food.

 A recent Canadian study found that women who eat peanuts have detectable amounts of peanut proteins in their breastmilk. If you have a history of nut allergies in your family, you may want to avoid nut products while you are breastfeeding.

Once you have identified a problem food, keep it off your menu for a few months. Older babies can more easily tolerate a variety of flavours. Another solution is to avoid large amounts of any one food at a time. Some women find that they are able to eat small amounts of their problem foods if they don't do it very often; however, no two women are the same, so you'll have to experiment a little.

Healthy Snacks

It's not always easy to prepare regular meals with a new baby in the house. Luckily, good nutrition is just as easy to achieve by 'grazing' as it is by eating three square meals every day. Keeping healthy snacks on hand is a great way to get your RDAs, keep off unwanted weight and set a good lifelong example for your child. Instead of crisps or biscuits, try some of the following quick and healthy alternatives or add your own from the Food Pyramid.

· Apples	· Cereal	· Popcorn (plain)
· Bananas	· Crackers	· Salads
· Breads	· Eggs	· Soups
· Canteloupe	· Grapes	· Strawberries
· Carrot sticks	· Oranges	· Tomatoes (may cause wind)
· Celery	· Plums	· Yogurt

Special Concerns

Whether you're a vegetarian or have medical restrictions, you'll want to take extra care. Special attention is important not only for your baby's nutrition, but also to preserve your own health. If you need additional information, consult your doctor or a nutritionist.

Vegetarian Diet

If you're a vegetarian, you already pay special attention to your diet. Lacto-ovo vegetarians, who eat eggs and dairy products, can generally meet all their nutritional needs from food sources. However, vegans, those vegetarians who don't eat any animal products at all, are at risk for nutritional deficiencies in several important areas. Protein, vitamin D, riboflavin, calcium, iron and zinc are harder to find in plant form than in animal products, but this can be done.

VITAMINS	
B_{12}	fortified soya beverages and cereals
D	fortified soya beverages and sunshine
Riboflavin (B_2)	fortified whole grains, avocados and nuts
MINERALS	
Calcium	soya beverages, calcium-enriched orange juice, broccoli, nuts, seeds, pak choi, greens, grains, peas and beans, kale and some tofus
Iron	green leafy vegetables, iron-fortified cereals and breads, peas, beans, tofu, dried fruits and whole grains
Zinc	tofu, nuts, peas, beans, wheatgerm, bran and wholewheat breads
PROTEINS	soya, nuts, seeds, peas, beans, grains and vegetables

Vitamin B_{12} does not naturally occur in plant sources, and vegans, lactating or not, need to supplement this important nutrient. Ask your health visitor for advice.

There is also some question about the availability of important, brain-nourishing fats such as DHA in strict vegan diets. Noted American paediatric experts Martha and William Sears believe so strongly in the importance of DHA in a breastfeeding woman's diet that they recommend that vegans temporarily add fish to their daily menu. Consider the following suggestions of good dietary sources for the nutrients most often lacking in vegetarian diets.

Teenage Mums

Mothers below the age of nineteen are still growing and have more nutritional needs than older mothers. Your health visitor or GP can advise you on special or additional dietary requirements. Phosphorus works with calcium to form teeth and bones. Magnesium is necessary in the production of healthy bones, teeth and nerves, and also helps prevent heart attacks and stroke. Teenage mothers should make special efforts to incorporate the following into their diet:

- Calcium: milk, cheese, whole grains, egg yolk, peas, beans, nuts, green leafy vegetables
- Phosphorus: milk, cheese, meat, egg yolk, whole grains, peas, beans, nuts
- Magnesium: dark green leafy vegetables, bananas, dried apricots, avocados, cashews, almonds, soya products, whole grains, chocolate

Weight-Loss Plans

Breastfeeding is a wonderful natural weight-loss plan. Studies consistently show that women who nurse their babies return to their pre-pregnancy weight faster than women who formula feed. All the fat cells your body stockpiled during pregnancy, and even some from before, will be used to make milk for your baby.

When you breastfeed, your body needs about 500 extra calories every day. That means you can eat a little bit more than usual and still lose weight. If you only consume an extra 300 calories every day, your body will use your fat stores to make up the difference.

Changes in your diet can pose a risk to your health if you have certain already existing medical conditions. If you are on a restricted diet of any kind, talk with your health-care provider before making any changes — even a vitamin and mineral pill can cause problems for some people.

Your weight loss while breastfeeding will be slow but steady; that's the way nature intended it. Crash dieting puts you at risk of nutritional deficiencies and might eventually affect the quality of your milk. Besides, crash diets don't work – studies show that rapid weight loss at any time of life is usually followed by rapid weight gain. The best way to keep weight off is to lose it gradually through a combination of diet and exercise.

Choosing healthy foods and drinking lots of water during lactation will get you into the right habits. Keep your weight loss down to 0.4kg (1lb) per week or less. Even half that amount per week will melt away that extra pregnancy weight within a year.

CHAPTER 15

Exercise for You and Your Baby

How can exercise affect breastfeeding? Anything that helps a nursing mother stay confident and ward off depression also helps her have a positive breastfeeding experience. Your mind and body have far-reaching effects on each other, and that connection can make all the difference in the quality of your life. It's vital to realize that exercise is not only compatible with lactation, it's beneficial as well.

The Benefits of Exercise

This might not feel like the best time to start or resume a programme of exercise, but exercise can help you in every part of your life, including breastfeeding. As little as 20–30 minutes of aerobic exercise three or four times per week can help you feel better, look better and live longer. Toning exercises such as sit-ups and leg lifts can help your body regain its pre-pregnancy shape more quickly. Any amount of exercise will burn up calories and help you lose some of that leftover pregnancy weight.

Exercise

·   Increases your energy level
·   Steps up your metabolism so you burn more calories, even at rest
·   Tones your muscles
·   Gives you a sense of accomplishment that boosts your confidence
·   Improves your circulation
·   Fights off depression and boredom
·   Helps you to lose weight
·   Makes you feel sexier

As important as exercise is, don't overdo it! Weight loss should be very gradual in breastfeeding women, otherwise you're putting yourself and your baby at risk for nutritional deficiencies. Exercise for health, not just weight loss. Ask your caregiver for advice.

Remember to always stretch before and after a workout. Stretching lengthens your muscles, increases your flexibility and greatly reduces your chance of injury. You'll also find stretching helpful in relieving muscle cramp and other muscle-related pains.

When to Begin

Always get your doctor's approval before beginning an exercise programme. There are conditions, like Caesarean section delivery and abdominal diastasis, that might keep you more sedentary than you would like. Adequate recovery time and sometimes specialized exercise routines are absolute necessities to avoid dangerous complications.

Doctors generally advise women without special conditions to wait at least six weeks after delivery before beginning or resuming an aerobic exercise programme. Your body needs the time both to recover from childbearing and to establish a good milk supply. You and your baby also need those first weeks to work out a nursing routine.

What is abdominal diastasis?
Labour can cause a separation of the vertical muscles in your abdomen, called diastasis, and even mild exertion can make it worse.

However, that doesn't mean you're on bed rest. Shaping and toning exercises are generally all right; sit-ups and leg lifts can help your body recover. You can also go about any normal activity that doesn't cause you pain or undue stress. Walking is a great all-around exercise at any time. Just take it slowly and work your way up to the level of activity you want.

Finding the Time

With all the new responsibilities of parenthood, clearing your schedule at a certain time every day for exercise isn't always practical. It's easy to get so busy that you forget to take care of yourself. Everyone else's needs seem to come first: your baby needs to be fed, changed and held; your toddler needs attention, stimulation and socialization; the dog needs to be walked. In those busy first months, you've got to become an exercise opportunist.

Make exercise part of your ordinary activities. Three 10-minute chunks of time are as effective as 30 minutes in one go. Shorter stretches are easier to get through and easier to schedule. Even little activities that seem as though they wouldn't make much of a difference add up quickly over the course of a few months.

· Sit up five or ten times in the morning when you first get out of bed. Add an extra sit-up every few days.

- Use the stairs instead of the lift.
- Park at the far end of the car park.
- Choose to stand instead of sit.
- Flex your muscles and hold them tight while you sit in traffic.
- Run in place.
- Tighten your pelvic floor muscles just about anywhere.
- Tackle the housework: washing, dishes, taking out the rubbish, washing windows and hoovering the floor are productive workouts.
- Do the garden work. Let your partner watch the baby while you weed, mow or shovel.

After you and your baby have worked out a sleep routine, you can start to enjoy more traditional workouts a few times per week. It's hard for new parents to imagine having the time for a formal workout, but remember that exercise only seems like it takes time; it really saves time. Ask a local sports centre if they run any classes especially designed for new mums – as well as being good for you, this is a great way to meet other new mothers.

Exercise sharpens both your mind and body, helping you cut through your tasks more quickly with less effort. The little bit of time you spend on exercise will pay you back many times over with increased efficiency.

Your Changing Body

During pregnancy, your body went through some major changes. Lactation adds new and different demands. Your body isn't the same as it was before pregnancy, and you've got to keep that in mind as you exercise.

1. Exercise regularly, at least three times per week. If you're playing a sport, don't compete.
2. Don't exercise too hard in hot, humid weather.
3. Keep your movements smooth. Don't bounce or jerk. Exercise on a wooden floor or a tightly carpeted surface.
4. Your joints are looser than normal, so avoid flexing or extending them very far. Loose joints can lead to dislocation or damage, so avoid jumping, jarring or rapid changes in direction.

5. Always warm up for five minutes before any vigorous workout; slow walking is a good warm-up.
6. At the end of a workout, slow down gradually and stretch. However, because your joints are looser than normal, don't stretch any joint to its maximum position.
7. Women should monitor their heart rates and stay within the range advised by their doctors.
8. Rise slowly. There's an increased risk of fainting due to sudden changes in your blood pressure. Work your legs gently for a few minutes after you get back on your feet.
9. Drink plenty of water to avoid dehydration. Drink whenever you're thirsty, even if it means interrupting the workout.
10. If you haven't been very active in the past, you should start slowly and increase your workout over time.
11. At the first sign of unusual symptoms, you should stop exercising and contact your doctor.

Lactating women need to take some other precautions as well. Nurse your baby or express your milk before working out and wear a good, supportive sports bra. Full breasts can be painful if they are jostled around too much.

After a workout, immediately remove your bra. Wash your breasts with plain water and let them air dry. A sweaty breast might be unappealingly salty to your baby, and clean, dry breasts are much less likely to become infected from clogged milk ducts.

Exercise and Breastmilk

Over the last few years, many of us have heard reports that exercise sours breastmilk and leads to fussy babies that reject the breast. This is simply not true: all the speculation is based on a single study that compared breastmilk samples taken before and after exhaustive exercise sessions.

In this study, it was observed that babies seemed less eager to take breastmilk immediately after their mothers had worked out to near exhaustion. Researchers blamed lactic acid, a normal by-product of exercise, for the effect. That's as much information as most of the public received. Less known is that the effect lasted for only about one hour. So if your exercise routine involves pushing on to the point of exhaustion, you might want to wait an hour before feeding your child. Otherwise, you really don't need to worry about any negative effects to your milk.

Exercises To Do with Your Baby

Involving your baby or toddler in your exercise routine makes working out fun, and it's a great way to get closer to your child.

- Put your baby in a sling or a buggy and go for a long family walk. You can walk through the park, around the shopping centre or just around your neighbourhood.
- Buy a jogging buggy with big bicycle tires and take your child on a run.
- Buy a bike trailer and take him for a ride.
- Pull your toddler behind you in a baby cart.
- Do sit-ups in front of your baby in a bouncy swing, and say 'peek-a-boo' every time you come forwards. She'll love it!
- Lie on the floor next to your baby and do leg lifts. It's a great way to exercise while still maintaining face-to-face contact.
- Dance with your child in your arms – this can be slow or fast or anywhere in between.
- Use your baby as a weight. When she is old enough to support her head, lift her up while you're lying on the floor. Bring her to your nose with a smile and some words of love, then put her back out at arm's length and do it again.

Toddlers can be a workout all by themselves – just try to keep up with yours for a while! If you really want a workout, take your toddler to the home of a friend who doesn't have children. People without kids always have lots of breakable things within a toddler's easy reach, and by the time you've followed two steps behind your curious youngster for an hour, you'll feel as if you've run a marathon.

CHAPTER 16

Stress, Postnatal Depression and Breastfeeding

Yes, your life has changed! Happy events such as moving or starting a new job can cause stress, and having a new baby is a major life adjustment. Learning to be the parent of a new baby might be both the happiest time in your life – as well as the most stressful. Now is the time to have friends and family present to share in this joyous time, and to support you in your new role.

'Discontented Cows Don't Give Milk'

I once spoke to the wife of a dairy farmer. She told me that dairy cows are made to feel as comfortable as possible in order to produce an abundant milk supply. They eat, sleep and give milk, and that's all that's expected of them. Don't all new mothers wish life were that simple! When women report problems relating to plugged ducts, mastitis and milk supply, in essence, that is the advice they are given – eat, sleep and give milk.

Stress and Your Milk Supply

Stress can affect your milk supply to some degree, but every woman is different. Some women who live in war-torn countries or who suffer from severe malnutrition can still supply enough milk to keep their babies well nourished. Other mothers don't fare as well. While the baby's demand will regulate your milk production, a stressed mother and a fretful baby are likely to threaten the success of the breastfeeding relationship.

Increased smoking and nicotine levels can have an impact on your milk supply. Smokers who are stressed tend to smoke more and inhale more deeply. If you are smoking more than a packet a day, you might experience a reduction in both your milk supply and your letdown.

Stress and fatigue cause an increase in adrenaline levels in the body, and adrenaline is a major inhibitor in the production of oxytocin, which commands the letdown reflex. When you're stressed, you may have a repressed letdown, which means that your baby must work harder to get milk from your breast. The harder he has to work, the more frustrated he becomes. This sets the stage for a difficult breastfeeding experience, and without intervention, it might end the beginning of a beautiful relationship.

An Ounce of Prevention

There are several ways to encourage relaxation and inner calm. One possible solution is creative visualization, which has been shown to improve milk supply. Camomile tea has been used for centuries as a mild sedative, and is safe for nursing women. Lavender oil on your pillowcase or massaged into your temples will help you relax and let your milk down. Breast massage before and during a feeding session is also beneficial.

Remember to nurse often and to focus on your baby. During the first few weeks, you're negotiating a nursing routine with your newborn, and frequent nursing will guarantee the maintenance of your milk supply. You might find breastfeeding stressful, but after your routine is established, it will be some of the best time you spend with your baby.

Sleep Deprivation

Being the parent of a newborn is like experiencing an altered state of consciousness. Many factors seem to work against your ability to get a good night's sleep: midnight feedings, regulating your sleep cycle to match your baby's, and recovering from labour anaesthesia all take their toll. Those stresses can create a surreal feeling of walking in a daze for those first few days after the birth of your infant.

Many experts, friends and family will tell new mothers to sleep when their baby sleeps. This piece of sage advice is priceless. Housework can wait, but your mental health cannot. Sleep as often as you can, or call a friend to babysit so you can rest soundly. Preserving your sleep time requires putting your baby to bed. Sometimes we are so caught up with gazing at their angelic faces in slumber that we hold them throughout their naps, but you'll have lots of opportunities to bond. For now, let sleeping babies lie. Other strategies include taking turns with your partner or assigning shifts at night.

The Baby Blues

In the 4th century, Hippocrates, the Father of Physicians, discovered a condition he called 'puerperal fever'. It was believed that 'suppressed lochial discharge' (the discharge following birth) inflamed the brain and caused delirium and manic attacks. An 11th-century female gynaecologist,

Trotula of Salerno, thought that 'if the womb is moist, the brain is filled with water, and the moisture running over the eyes compels women to involuntarily shed tears'. Even in the 18th century, a book by a physician named Marcé was entitled *Treatise on Insanity in Pregnant and Lactating Women*. Although these physicians were onto something, their definitions were scientifically suspect and politically incorrect by today's standards. In the spirit of the day, however, this was an important acknowledgment that the baby blues is a very real condition.

Some 50–90 per cent of women experience some form of the baby blues. These tearful, weepy days usually begin about three to five days following birth, as hormones rapidly change in response to the loss of the placenta. Sleep deprivation, lack of confidence in parenting a newborn, isolation from the outside world and the 24/7 demands of a new baby serve only to compound these feelings.

How can hypothyroidism affect your milk supply?
Hypothyroidism occurs when the thyroid gland fails to produce a sufficient amount of its hormone. This hormone regulates your metabolism and can cause a reduction in your milk supply. Symptoms can include nervousness, sweating, increased heart palpitations, upset stomach, diarrhoea and weight loss. A physical examination by your doctor will diagnose or rule out this condition in relationship to postnatal depression.

The blues are characterized by feelings of inadequacy, exhaustion, confusion, euphoria, insomnia and mood swings. Because the vast majority of women experience some of these symptoms, this condition is considered normal. The baby blues are also considered transient: these feelings usually disappear within the first two weeks following birth, and sometimes they go away within hours of when they began.

Most women tend to muddle through, have a good cry to release some tension, or seek support from a strong husband or good friend. However, if your mood doesn't improve by the time your baby is two weeks old, or if your feelings seem overwhelming, tell your health-care provider. He or she might provide some additional testing or refer you to a counsellor. The baby blues can lead to postnatal depression (PND), a much more serious condition.

Stress-Stopping Toolbox

Things that seem so obvious are truly innovative for new, breastfeeding mothers engrossed in taking care of their babies. Ways to relax and take care of yourself may be the furthest thing from your mind, but remember that your physical and mental health is critical to successful breastfeeding and parenting. With this in mind, remember to do or get at least a few of the following every day:

Breathe. Lie on your bed and take deep abdominal cleansing breaths. Focus on your breathing. Try yoga.

Eat right and eat light. High-protein foods such as nuts, seeds and beans will increase your energy level. So will iron-rich foods such as eggs, red meat, fish, poultry, wholegrain cereals and breads, dried fruits and legumes. Drink a glass of orange juice with these; vitamin C helps your body absorb iron more efficiently. Iron will help you combat fatigue and anaemia. Prepare handy bags of baby carrots or grapes. They'll be ready when you are for a quick snack break.

Exercise. Your body releases endorphins after several minutes of exercise. Endorphins are your body's natural painkillers; they also make you feel good about yourself and are considered a natural high. Put your newborn in a buggy and walk around the block.

Laugh. Rent a funny film, read a humorous book or talk to a friend who makes you giggle. Laughter is indeed the best medicine.

Massage. A good massage reduces the stress hormone known as cortisol. It also boosts your immune system, alleviates stress, helps you relax and induces sleep. And it feels so good! Long, slow strokes that follow the growth of hair follicles (downward motions) relax the body, while strokes that go against hair growth (upward motions) stimulate your body. Always remember to avoid direct pressure on the spine when giving massage.

Prioritize. Is it more important to take care of yourself or your washing? This is a very busy time for you. Think about what really matters most. Now that you are a family, work may have to wait. Don't let someone else's crisis be your own. Slow down and reprioritize your goals.

Find a babysitter so you can go to the cinema, take a walk, read a book or go shopping. Do those things you enjoyed before your baby arrived. You need time to re-energize yourself, too!

Sleep. There is no better way to re-energize than to take catnaps whenever possible. Sleep when your baby sleeps; or better yet, lie down together and breastfeed. Develop bedtime rituals for yourself and your baby: bath, book, bed. As a new parent, you probably won't have any trouble falling asleep, but if you do, try eating healthy bedtime snacks that induce sleep, such a slice of chicken on a bagel with a glass of warm milk.

Take vitamins. Your prenatal vitamins contain minerals such as magnesium, folic acid and zinc. Those, coupled with B and C vitamins, will help maintain your body's energy. Vitamins alone can't accomplish what a healthy, balanced diet can, so use them in conjunction with nutritious foods.

Talk. Your frustrations are real. Call a friend, a parent or a crisis line, if needed. Join a parents' group or an Internet chat line for new parents. Develop new support systems with people who have previous experience in parenting. Surround yourself with positive people.

Try black walnuts. Black walnut teas, supplements and meats boost serotonin levels and combat depression.

Use aromatherapy. Add a few drops of jasmine, clary sage, lavender or rose oil to your bath or bed pillow. These scents have been shown to reduce stress and induce relaxation.

Walk. Fresh air can work wonders for a distressed spirit.

Taking care of yourself sometimes means simply going easy on yourself. Be mindful of your expectations, especially the universal one: somehow you will be the perfect parent. As you know, no one is perfect and no one can do it all, at least not for long. Don't set yourself up to fail, and don't sweat over the small details. Realistic expectations can decrease your risk for PND and relieve your anxiety.

Postnatal Depression

When the baby blues extends beyond what is considered the normal two-week period, it may turn into a more serious condition called postpartum depression, or PND.

· PND affects 10–30 per cent of all new mothers. The number of teenage and single parents with this condition is even higher.
· If left untreated, 25 per cent of women will still suffer from the symptoms up to one year later.
· The onset of PND usually occurs within the first six weeks after birth.

PND is characterized by feelings of listlessness, frequent crying, insomnia, anger, sadness, headaches, anxiety attacks and a sense of hopelessness. Take the quiz below to see how you score on the scale.

Postnatal Depression Quiz

Since the birth of your baby, have you experienced...

❑ Loss of interest in usually pleasurable activities?
❑ Difficulty concentrating or making decisions?
❑ Changes in appetite and/or sleep?
❑ Excessive anxiety over your baby's health?
❑ Feelings of worthlessness or guilt, especially feelings of failure as a mother?
❑ Fatigue?
❑ Excessive, repetitive or nervous non-productive activity such as pacing, fidgeting or an inability to sit still?
❑ A lack of desire to care for yourself, your infant or your family?
❑ Recurrent thoughts of death or suicide?

If you answered yes to four or more of these questions, you could be diagnosed as having PND. Contact your health-care provider immediately and take this test with you. You don't have to feel alone. There is help available right now!

What Causes PND and How Is It Treated?

No one is certain what causes PND, but most experts agree that many factors play a role.

During pregnancy, hormones such as oestrogen, progesterone, prolactin and cortisol, as well as ovarian steroids, interact to maintain a healthy pregnancy. After the delivery of the placenta, these hormone levels rapidly decline. Some alter central nervous system responses such as memory, movement, language, emotions, thought processes and involuntary body processes. The central nervous system is also important in the regulation of attention, sleep and arousal.

There is also a clear connection between a family history of depression and PND. If you have previously been diagnosed with depression, tell your doctor. The risk of having PND with a second baby is one hundred times greater if you've had it before.

Women with poor or abusive relationships, who lack support and suffer child-care stress have an increased risk of PND. Women with prior histories of depression, panic disorder, obsessive-compulsive disorder, premenstrual syndrome or previous PND episodes are at the greatest risk. Notify your health-care provider immediately.

PND is generally treated in three phases. Medications such as Zoloft, Prozac, Paxil or tricyclic antidepressants, safe for breastfeeding mothers, are widely used to treat symptoms in the first six to 12 weeks following diagnosis. Tricyclic antidepressants are commonly used with lactating women because there are fewer side effects in the infants of treated mothers. Prozac can cause some weight loss and takes longer for your body to shed, so this is a medication used as a last resort, but it's still possible to nurse while taking this drug.

Multiple births present increased challenges to your mental health. With the loss of their one supersized placenta or two smaller ones, mothers of multiples experience a more massive shift in hormones than other mothers. This puts them at a greater risk for PND.

Although PND is a serious condition, it is treatable. The condition itself is outside your control, but you do have control to take steps towards recovery. You're not alone and shouldn't have to suffer by yourself. Contact mental health professionals in your community who specialize in postnatal disorders. Call your health visitor of GP for referrals to individuals who can assist you. Remember, seeking help when you need it is a sign of strength, not a weakness.

PND and Breastfeeding

When diagnosed with PND, many women are told to wean their babies in order to be treated with antidepressants, but this is not always the best course of action. Weaning can compound feelings of depression by further reducing your body's production of prolactin. In fact, in many women, symptoms of PND don't appear until weaning begins.

Prolactin is the hormone responsible for initiating milk production. It's also nature's built-in tranquillizer for nursing mothers. Prolactin levels in your body increase when your baby suckles. Perhaps not coincidentally, PND is often diagnosed at six weeks post partum, the time when many women must return to work and have prepared to end their exclusive breastfeeding relationship.

Some depressed mothers often fail to respond appropriately to their infant's cues to feed, or might allow others to offer formula because they are simply not motivated to breastfeed. Each of these situations can have devastating effects on both your infant and your milk supply. Babies of depressed mothers sometimes develop depression, too. Seek assistance from your health-care provider if you suspect your baby might be affected by your depression.

Studies indicate that women who have active support present during their labour and delivery have fewer reported episodes of PND. Although some women might have more support at home than you have, there are steps you can take to enjoy a less stressful labour and delivery: doulas, partners, family and friends are all available to make your birthing experience a more positive one.

If you've been diagnosed with PND, you can continue to breastfeed. As long as your medications are safe, you can nurse your baby. Your doctor will prescribe the minimum effective dose and will monitor your infant throughout the process.

Resources for PND

Make sure to tell your health-care provider if your baby blues extend beyond the first two weeks after your baby's birth. Their goal is to develop a health history with you, so they need to know what sources of support are available and what services you've tried.

Your midwife, health visitor or GP are a good first port of call, and in addition the following organizations can provide support and advice:

NHS Direct	0845 464748
Association for Postnatal Illness	020 7386 0868
MIND (National Association for Mental Health)	08457 660163
National Childbirth Trust (NCT)	08704 448707
MAMA (Meet-a-Mum Association)	01761 433598
SANELINE	08457 678000

Support from Family and Friends

In many cultures, extended family and women relatives attend the birth of the baby, then keep watch over mother and infant for 30 days following delivery, and sometimes longer. This kith-and-kin network offers parents a chance to get to know their babies without the stress of having to do all the chores of life, such as preparing meals and house cleaning.

The Western Way

The extended family socialization of other cultures has worked for centuries for many reasons. In addition to the 'many hands make light work' element, friends and family provide much-needed emotional support for new parents. These communities have fewer reported cases of PND because they offer support throughout the time when family adjustment is most critical.

In our society, we operate a little differently. While mothers and mothers-in-law often come to stay for a week or so, women feel more inclined to entertain them as guests, rather than to accept their assistance. If this is the case for you, it is important to limit the number of visitors who come to call during the first few weeks after your baby arrives. If you have a hard time saying no, ask your partner to check your phone calls, or simply say, 'I'd like to have you over once things settle down a bit. I appreciate your patience and look forward to seeing you.'

Use Your Resources

If you can truly use the support your friends offer, then by all means accept it. There are several different types of support, and we need them all: emotional, informational, tangible and social.

Knowledge is power – Informational support is the easiest to access. When we have questions, we read a book, search the Web, call an expert or ask a friend. However, other types of support can be more difficult to obtain.

Open up! – Sharing intimate moments with people who care about you and understand you facilitates emotional support. Your partner, best friend and family are there for you, to listen and provide advice and encouragement. This kind of support is extremely valuable if you suffer from symptoms of PND or stress. Your loved ones genuinely want to help and will be there when you call.

Gift horses – Tangible support comes by way of baby-sitting offers, nappies and supplies, cash assistance or lifts to the supermarket. There might be times when this help is desperately needed. Keep these offers open-ended for when they come in handy.

Network – Social support includes groups of people who can provide assistance in a general way, such as your health-care provider, La Leche League and your colleagues and other acquaintances. The help they offer can take the form of participation in groups and programmes, or individual services based on your particular needs.

Asking for support takes a certain amount of bravery, but it will come more easily each time your call is answered. Concentrate on one helper with one task for one time. The goal is to seek assistance over the first few weeks of your baby's life.

What can a man do if his partner suffers from PND?
Your patience and encouragement are loving ways to communicate your support for her. Listen to her feelings and try to understand her. Don't blame her for something outside of her control. Take care of your baby as best you can, and don't ignore your own feelings – you are important, too!

Remember, too, that relationships are based on give and take. After your life has settled down and you are in a comfortable routine, you can pay back these favours one at a time. Most people find great satisfaction in helping others. Welcome the chance to return favours when the time comes.

CHAPTER 17

Sex and the Breastfeeding Couple

Western culture loves to emphasize the sexuality of the breasts. Conversely, some people, even health-care professionals, want to desexualize the breast entirely. They point out that breasts are clearly designed to feed babies, and that's serious business. Your breasts are wonderful sources of nourishment and emotional comfort for your baby, but they're sexual, too. Your challenge is to find the balance that works for you and your partner.

The Great Sexuality Debate

People who want to desexualize breasts are usually reacting to the way sexuality can interfere with breastfeeding. For instance, some men find it difficult at first to share their partner's breasts with a baby. They might be unwilling to accommodate any other use for their private playground. It seems as if everything from public nursing to our most private thoughts and feelings about breastfeeding can get completely tangled up in our attitudes to sex.

Let's say right here that, yes, breasts are sexual – but your whole body is sexual. When it comes to making a body part sexual, it's in the way that you use it. In many cultures, breasts are just one more piece of a woman's anatomy, such as an arm or a leg. There are cultures (and individuals) that find a well-turned ankle, the eyes or even a quick mind far more exciting than an exposed breast.

Do some women feel aroused while breastfeeding?
It's normal for some women to become sexually aroused while breastfeeding. Oxytocin, the hormone released by your body when baby suckles, is also released during sex. Some women even reach orgasm. Breastfeeding is a pleasurable experience. It's one of nature's rewards.

Speaking of minds, the brain is your most important sexual organ. Sex is a combination of friction and fantasy. For some men, part of the thrill of breasts is the context in which they have access to them. If your partner is one of these men, he might only be used to seeing your breasts during sexual encounters.

So, now are your breasts only for the baby? No, not if you're comfortable with breast play as a part of your sexual relationship with your partner. Your breasts can be less sensitive, oversensitive or unchanged in the weeks following birth. All these conditions are normal. If you enjoy the contact, there's no reason you can't resume breast play.

Changing Relationships

Before your baby was born, the relationship you enjoyed with your partner took centre stage in your life. You were lovers, friends and playmates. Now, you're parents. For some people, it's difficult to reconcile these new roles with the old ones. Some men believe that their partner's new status as mother makes her untouchable.

Men like that need a little reminder that their partners are still sexual beings. Are mothers sexy? Of course they are! Mothers are women, not girls. They have given birth. They're fertile and sensuous. If you're ready for sex but your partner doesn't seem interested, make the first move. Most men love that. It might be just the thing he needs to jog his memory about how you became parents in the first place.

tips

Most women experience a lack of interest in sex following the birth of their baby. Hormonal changes serve to focus a new mother's attention where nature wants it, on the baby. It's a temporary condition, but combined with sleep deprivation, it can leave little room for romance.

Nursing your baby is a wonderfully satisfying, intimate experience. You might even come to feel that your body belongs first to your baby, and second to your partner. Your hormone levels while lactating can contribute to those feelings. Oestrogen levels are low, and that affects your desire for sex as well as the amount of natural lubrication produced by your vagina. It's as if nature were saying, 'You've got a baby. You don't need sex until it's time for another one.'

Although your sexual needs might have temporarily changed, your partner's needs are nearly the same as they've always been. He might be a little less amorous than usual because of the exhaustion that's common to all new parents, but he still looks forward to spending time alone with you. That doesn't mean you have to supply him with sex on demand, just try to stay connected emotionally. One way is to keep your partner involved in your most important activity, the care of your child.

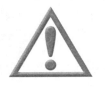

You might not feel that your partner knows what he's doing when he tries to help out, but resist the urge to correct your partner when he changes a nappy or attempts to comfort your crying child. It's vital that your partner bonds with your baby, too. You're not just nurturing a child, you're nurturing a family.

Just for Dads

The two of you are in this thing together, and you need each other now more than you ever have before. Your lives have changed, and they won't be getting back to 'normal'. It's up to you and your partner to find a new 'normal' for your relationship. Give her the support she needs to be a good mother. If you find yourself doing more around the house, don't think in terms of 'I'm helping her out' – your life together is a partnership. Court her to remind her that she's the love of your life. A loving relationship with your partner is one of the best gifts you can give your baby. Stay intimate in a hundred little ways, and don't pressure her for sex, as you'll both feel bad about it later.

Intimacy

Intimacy doesn't mean sex. Rather, true intimacy is a matter of the mind. It's simply knowing and caring about your partner's thoughts, needs and feelings, but mostly it's about trust: trust that you'll be there when you're needed; trust that you'll love your partner no matter what; and trust that you can be yourself with each other. The two of you are a team.

Where there's true intimacy between a couple, sex follows naturally. Until you're both ready for physical intimacy, you can stay connected with your partner in many simple, non-sexual ways.

· Leave love notes around the house for your partner.
· Take a walk together.
· Surprise your partner with a gift. It doesn't have to be anything big, just a little way of saying, 'I'm thinking of you'.

- Say 'I love you' and mean it.
- Go out. Take a deep breath and hire that babysitter. Go to your favourite restaurant or have a picnic. It's all right to talk about the baby – it might be hard to think about anything else at first. Your child is the focus of your life right now, but don't let that one topic dominate the conversation.
- Laugh together.
- Help out around the house.
- Take an interest in the activities your partner enjoys.
- Give a massage. A breastfeeding mum is especially prone to sore back and shoulders. You can even rub her feet while she nurses the baby.
- Look your best. Often you just need to be comfortable around your home and joggers and a T-shirt are fine. On occasion, though, treat your partner to the glamorous version of you that's usually reserved for special events. Making yourself attractive for your partner shows them how important they are to you.
- Write a love song or rewrite the words to an existing song. Your song can be dripping with romance or it can be funny. As an alternative, make a tape or CD of the songs that are special to the two of you.
- Give up some minor habit you know annoys your partner. Tapping your fingers or putting your elbows on the table may seem minor issues, but changing your behaviour out of love is a major gesture.

Through it all, communicate. Talk about everything. It's especially important to discuss your feelings before a problem develops. Use the phrase 'I feel…' instead of assuming that your feelings are an accurate measure of the situation.

If you can communicate openly and respectfully with each other, you'll find that you share many of the same thoughts and fears. Together, you can reach much more mutually satisfying solutions than you ever could apart. Keeping the lines of communication open will even help with those situations where all you can do is endure. Labour, exhaustion, colic and a new parent's fears are all easier to take when you have a hand to hold and a shoulder to cry on.

Sex

Basically the time to resume your sex life is when you both want to – there is no 'right' or 'wrong' time. In any case, your body needs some time to heal. The separation in your uterine lining caused by the expulsion of the placenta must close and tears or episiotomy incisions have to heal and become flexible again.

Numbers and norms vary among women, but research has clearly shown that breastfeeding speeds recovery from pregnancy and childbirth. A faster recovery would seem to naturally favour a more immediate return to sexual readiness.

Breastfeeding may also have an influence on how quickly women resume sex, but it's difficult to tell based on current research. One study reported that breastfeeding couples tend to wait a little longer than other couples. Another study reported that breastfeeding mothers not only resumed sexual relations sooner after birth than other mothers, but enjoyed it more and experienced less pain. In agreement, yet another study suggests that women who breastfeed return to arousability sooner than women who don't breastfeed.

The Big Day

Eventually you'll feel ready for intercourse. That first time after childbirth can be a lot like your other first time – the experience can be anywhere from mildly uncomfortable to downright painful. When you're ready to give it a try, you'll need to take a few special precautions.

Relax. In her popular book, *The Girlfriends' Guide to Surviving the First Year of Motherhood*, Vicki McCarty Lovine recommends that you 'inebriate and lubricate'. That advice might work for some women, but breastfeeding mothers need to be careful about using a glass of wine or any other alcoholic beverage to help them relax. Whenever you plan to have a drink, nurse your baby first and allow at least one hour to pass for every drink you consume before breastfeeding your baby again. If you feed your baby and then have two glasses of wine, you should wait at least two hours from the last drink. Most new mothers are exhausted, and alcohol can send them right to sleep.

Pay attention to lubrication. Post-partum oestrogen levels reduce your vagina's natural lubrication, so have a tube of the artificial stuff on hand. K-Y jelly is a good choice, and spermicidal jellies are another. Normal amounts of lubrication usually return after your first menstrual cycle.

Use birth control. You might need to try a different method from usual while breastfeeding. Consult the sections on fertility and birth control below for advice.

Take the lead. Women generally prefer to be on top or lie side-by-side with their partner (the spoon position) during intercourse. These positions let you control the amount of pressure put on delicate perineal tissue.

Communicate. Women, let your partner know what you enjoy and what's just too uncomfortable right now; don't suffer through the event. Your partner wants you to enjoy yourself. That might be a tall order the first few times, but at a minimum, you shouldn't have to be in pain. If you decide to grin and bear it, you're just going to be even more nervous about sex in the future, and this can lead to a loss of intimacy with your partner if you become afraid that loving attention will lead to another painful sexual encounter.

Expect some milk leakage. Sexual stimulation releases oxytocin, the hormone that causes your milk ejection, or letdown, reflex. Your breasts might leak when you make love and even spray your partner in the face when you orgasm. If that's a problem (and who says it has to be?), nurse your baby before you have sex, or wear a bra and nursing pads. In any case, you'll want to keep a towel handy – these things are loaded, and they might just go off!

Take your time. It's been a while, but a new mum's body is too sensitive to rush things. Dad, you've waited this long; a few more minutes won't hurt. Foreplay should be long and relaxed.

Men, don't feel that you absolutely have to finish what you've started. If you're at home, your baby might cry right in the middle of the event you've waited so patiently for. It's not anybody's fault. This is one of those times when you have to switch gears from 'lover' to 'father' so quickly you might feel as if you've left your transmission lying somewhere along the road. If you want to score a few points towards the next time, go and get the baby and bring her to your wife to nurse.

Golden Opportunities

Once you've broken the ice that first time, you'll need to find more time for romance in the future. This may sound like Mission Impossible, but you can plan for those special times with your partner. Just stay as rested as you can, and keep a record of the times during the day and night when your baby is blissfully asleep. These are your opportunities!

It can take anywhere from a few weeks to an entire year for sex to become as comfortable as it was before pregnancy. Then you'll face a whole new set of challenges. Your child is mobile. If you make love when she's awake, she will find you: toddlers are like bloodhounds.

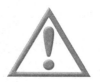

It's absolutely vital that you do not leave your toddler unattended for more than a minute or two. If you must be away from her, remove any hazards from the room and take along the baby monitor. It only takes moments for tragedy to strike an active child.

Once again, it's time to get creative – you've got to take the opportunity for sex when you can get it. If your child loves a certain TV show, that might be your chance. Although you might dislike him now, you may one day be grateful for Bob the Builder.

Even after your toddler has settled into a bigger bed, you're not safe. Toddlers still tend to walk right in on you in the middle of things, so keep the bedroom door closed, but don't lock it. This won't help: there's nothing like your child yelling for mummy outside the door to put an end to the mood. Just be ready to assume a casual position and have a plausible story prepared for when you're caught.

Your Body

The weeks and months following the birth of your baby are a time of transition for your body. Internally, your uterus, cervix and vagina are recovering. Breastfeeding helps – when your baby nurses, you will feel your uterus contract. At first it can hurt, but after the uterus regains its normal size, those contractions often become pleasurable.

Pelvic floor exercises are a great way to firm the muscles in the pelvic floor. Do them as often as you can. To make sure you're doing it right, occasionally practice while you're urinating.

1. Tense up your vaginal and anal muscles as if you were trying to stop a stream of urine.
2. Hold the tension for five seconds.
3. Relax and repeat three to five times.

Like your uterus, your vagina was stretched by childbirth. Many women worry that their vaginas will never regain their predelivery size and wonder if their husbands will find sex less satisfying than before. However, the vagina is a truly remarkable organ – it can expand to accommodate a baby's head and then shrink back to its normal size in just a few days. If you want to accelerate the process, just tighten your pelvic muscles; pelvic floor exercises are very effective.

Men, you may really enjoy some of the changes in your wife's body. Remember, there's only one right answer to the question 'How do I look?' That answer is 'Beautiful'. Disparaging comments about your mate's body, even in jest, can destroy the intimacy your relationship needs to last the test of time. A mother's body isn't the body of a girl. It's a woman's body – fuller, softer, and more sensuous.

On the other hand, don't go overboard praising your lover's new looks. For example, if you enjoy her somewhat enhanced cleavage too much, she'll come to believe that her non-lactating breasts are less desirable.

Fertility and Milk Production

Breastfeeding is nature's own form of birth control. If you exclusively breastfeed your baby, you are unlikely to be fertile. A drop in oestrogen production is one of the hormonal changes necessary for milk production to begin, and this results in reduced fertility. Doctors call this lactational amenorrhoea. Your menstrual cycle stops, and your fertility is so drastically cut that it's like you're using the contraceptive pill. For a woman with lactational amenorrhoea, there's less than a 2 per cent chance of conception.

Despite this remarkable contraceptive power, most authorities advise women to use an additional form of birth control to be safe. The reason behind this recommendation is simple: lactational amenorrhoea is easily interrupted, and you might ovulate before the return of your menses. Some women are simply caught off guard.

Birth Control

You need to be aware of the impact other contraceptive methods may have on your breastfeeding experience and, possibly, your baby. The safest choice while nursing is a method that doesn't involve chemicals – this means natural family planning, condoms, diaphragms and cervical caps. The next best choices are products using spermacides, such as foams, gels and sponges.

Avoid contraceptive pills that are high in oestrogen, which can reduce your milk production. The more common progestin-only pills are considered safe for breastfeeding mothers, as are progestin injections or subdermal implants. For breastfeeding women, injections such as Depo-Provera are slightly less effective than implants such as Norplant. Although hormonal steroids have not been shown to pose any risk to your baby, they do pass into your milk in small amounts. Some health-care professionals worry about early exposure of infants to these compounds and advise breastfeeding women to delay their use.

Talk to your doctor for more information about birth control options.

CHAPTER 18
Siblings and Family Life

magine this: one day your partner arrives home with another woman. 'Darling, I love you so much, I wanted another one just like you. I will be spending most of my time with her, but you'll grow to love her and she'll be a great addition to our family.' Now imagine what a child would feel if you brought a new baby home without taking steps to help her prepare emotionally.

Family Transitions

New babies are big adjustments, and children experience a wide variety of reactions based on their age and maturity levels. There may be some regression, such as bed-wetting or loss of interest in potty training. Toddlers might want to taste breastmilk or suck on a bottle, even after they've been weaned from both. There may be feelings of excitement, anger or sadness, and often all three.

It takes time for feelings to surface, and young children often don't have the words to express them once they do; sometimes the feelings are just too big for words. All of these reactions are normal, and the best way to deal with them is to prepare well in advance.

Toddlers (Age One to Three)

Toddlers are busy, independent, mobile, curious, active and often oblivious to the fact that a new baby is in the house, unless it somehow affects their agenda or their possessions. Most parents of toddlers know the Toddler Law of Property by now: 'What's mine is mine and what's yours is mine, unless it's broken, then it's yours, but all the small pieces I can choke on are still mine.'

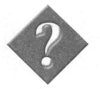

What is common regressive behaviour in toddlers?
Clinging, whining, crying, bed-wetting and waking at night are common regressive patterns. All these reactions are normal, but patience will see you through. Children should not be punished or rewarded for regressive behaviour – ignore the things you can, and be patient with the rest.

The Toddler Law of Property applies to you, too. You belong to your toddler, and there will be some level of jealousy with limited lap time and attention. Your toddler is used to being the baby and to being treated as such. The shift from 'baby' to 'big brother or sister' is a change of status that can leave your toddler feeling displaced.

Make arrangements for your toddler to stay with a nurturing adult while you're in hospital. Toddlers have difficulty with abrupt transitions and often suffer from separation anxiety; it's best to prepare early and to make their stay sound like an adventure. Once you're admitted to hospital, make frequent phone calls to check on her – she needs to hear your voice and know that you'll come back soon. Don't forget to pack her lovies, such as a favourite blanket or stuffed animal. These are useful transitional objects that keep her connected to you while you're physically apart.

Sexual Education

You've entered the 'why' stage of parenting. When answering toddler questions, it's important to keep your answers simple, short, age-appropriate and honest. It's easy to overload a toddler who wants only his specific question answered; others will follow, that's for certain, and you may be answering the same question in several different, yet creative, ways. Always focus on one question at one time.

Your toddler may take an interest in breastfeeding, too. After the birth of her baby brother, four-year-old Jennifer asked her mother, Linda, if she could have a taste of breastmilk. Linda allowed it, and Jennifer never asked again. When Suzanne nursed Ian, Meaghan would grab her doll, lift her shirt and 'nurse' her baby. These are important lessons in both nutrition and nurturing, as well as positive female role modelling. Young girls turn into grown-up women, and they need to know the rules of the game.

Toolbox Tricks

Toddlers benefit from learning about babies by observing them in action. Before your baby is born, invite friends with infants to visit you so your toddler can explore and learn about gentle touch. Toddlers continue to learn best through sensory contact, so touch, taste, sight, smell and hearing are important teaching strategies to use.

When your new baby comes home with you, explore her together. Count fingers and toes. Touch her skin. Allow your toddler to hold the baby with supervision.

When it's time to nurse, have a basket full of toys, books, crayons, envelopes, stickers, junk mail and flyers, paper and interesting household items handy. Get it out only when you breastfeed, as this gives the basket a special meaning. Have snacks ready, too – children will often wait until your newborn has latched on perfectly and is nursing contentedly to ask for a drink or a snack. If you keep nutritious snacks and juice cartons in your basket, they'll be ready when you need them.

Like the rest of us, toddlers have good and not-so-good days. Accept these feelings and remember that they are often short-lived. Parents of toddlers know that mood dictates behaviour. Anticipate when they'll need a nap or a snack, and meet their needs before major ructions occur.

If you have a sling, you can nurse your newborn baby as you take your toddler for a walk around the block. With time, you'll learn how to nurse one-handed. You can use the other hand to hold your toddler or help turn the pages of a storybook.

Preschool Children (Age Three to Five)

It's difficult to predict how your preschool child will react to your new baby. When visiting you and your new addition in the hospital, most children of this age will take little interest in the baby and will be more curious about how high the hospital bed can go or whether they can keep the bendy straws in the cup.

Don't expect immediate bonding between siblings, and don't be surprised if there's a complete lack of interest from your child. This doesn't mean jealousy. As new parents, we're on guard to protect our children from feeling emotions we label as negative, but having those feelings are an important part of growing up.

Sexual Education

Preschool children have a natural curiosity about their bodies and those of their friends. This is the 'doctor' stage of development, when children can identify themselves and their peers as girls or boys and are entering a sexual identity stage. They explore their bodies enthusiastically and know what makes them feel good. Pregnancy and birth are excellent times to begin light sexual education with your preschool child. Again, answers should be short and sweet. Give real names to body parts, and refer to your breasts as 'breasts' and not 'boobies'.

Three-year-olds are often fascinated by the nappy change of a baby of the opposite gender; this experience provides golden opportunities to talk about body parts and sexual differences in a healthy way. Defining sexual organs by their appropriate names sets the stage for healthy sexual identity now and later in life.

Toolbox Tricks

Preschool children love books. A trip to the library to gather books about newborn care is a helpful way to introduce your new baby. Choose books with lots of photographs.

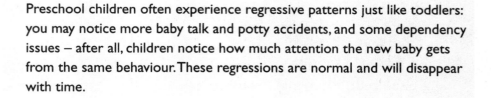

fact

Preschool children often experience regressive patterns just like toddlers: you may notice more baby talk and potty accidents, and some dependency issues – after all, children notice how much attention the new baby gets from the same behaviour. These regressions are normal and will disappear with time.

Preschool children love art as well, and will create 'elaborate' drawings of a circle head and stick legs to represent a person. More advanced artists might include stick arms and eyeballs, but that's usually only on request. You can extend a drawing session while you're nursing by asking your preschool child to add facial features, clothing, accessories, action and background. A basket of coloured pencils, crayons, blank paper, notebooks and colouring books should hold their interest for the length of a feeding session.

Teach your preschool child the art of hand massage. Make this her important job with the new baby, and let her know you appreciate her help in the caregiving role.

Ask your preschool child to share stories about her new brother or sister. Those stories are often heavily veiled discussions about their own feelings and private thoughts – help them find the words and meanings.

How can I be sure my preschool child has enough time with children his own age?
Schedule play dates with other children or enroll in a half-day early education programme. Socialization with same-aged peers is important for your preschool child, and gives you special time alone with your newborn.

School-Aged Children (Age Five to Twelve)

School-aged children are often enthusiastic and excited about having a new baby in the house. They are busy with school, friends and outside activities, and often view a new baby as a novelty.

Older children approach babies playfully. They model parenting skills, too. It's sometimes like watching a reflection of yourself as they coo and cuddle with their new infant. Be proud that you've taught them well.

School-aged children are good at discussing their feelings, especially around bedtime, so make your routines with them sacred. There is something magical about the bedtime hour that makes kids open up: it's dim and intimate, and communication flows. It might simply be that your children don't want to go to sleep, but regardless of your child's motivation, take advantage of these opportunities by sharing feelings. Listen with an open mind and an open heart.

Sexual Education

This is the stage where children think kissing is yucky, and at the same time it is when they notice the amount of sex used in advertising and magazines. It is an excellent time to have a discussion about the birds and the bees, if your child is interested and you're comfortable with the topic. As with children of any age, it's important not to overload them with information; it may be helpful finding out what they already know and building on that.

Breastfeeding gives children a healthy view of the human body. It also demonstrates the natural use of the breast. Children who grow up in breastfeeding homes are often more comfortable about their own bodies and sexual identities than those who don't.

Children on the school playground are like a trainee secret society. They've shared secrets about how babies are made, as well as dispelled myths about the tooth fairy and other mystical gift-givers. However, there is a lot of misinformation out there – children who don't know all the answers often speculate and fill in the blanks with something shocking or downright hilarious.

Toolbox Tricks

Ask your school-aged child to write a letter to the new baby welcoming her home. Take a picture of your new baby so Dad can pack it in the lunch box as a surprise. Because breastfed babies are extremely mobile, ask your child if he would like you to stay with the new baby in the school playground at collection time so that his friends can also see her.

School-aged children still need to spend quality time with you. Make arrangements for Dad to stay with smaller children as you and your Year 4 child go out for ice-cream. Ask your child to plan a special one-on-one activity for an afternoon out.

School-aged children are great entertainers. Get them to try these games with your new baby to make her laugh: hold a silly face contest, play tickle games, recite 'This Little Piggy', play peek-a-boo, play puppets, make animal sounds or blow bubbles. Involve the whole family in entertainment!

Preserve routines as much as possible: children need stability, security and the ability to predict the day's events. They also need a good night's sleep and healthy snacks and meals. Too many changes too quickly can leave everyone in turmoil. Patience and planned transition time will help smooth the way for major changes in your family's life.

Teenagers (Thirteen and Over)

Eeewwww. Enough said? You had sex, and your teenager is mortified that someone your age still engages in such activities. On top of that, you're breastfeeding: you've bared your breasts in front of other people when your teenager thinks you should be hiding in a cupboard; teenagers might not be used to seeing breasts (other than a quick glance at their own) outside PG movies. In addition, their own emerging sexuality makes it difficult to think about their parents in sexual terms.

Teens have entered a very dramatic period in their lives, when their hormones play an important role in their behaviour. They are often emotional, easily embarrassed, moody, withdrawn and private. They're working on acquiring grown-up skills while coming to terms with their own changing bodies – and sometimes their bodies are maturing more quickly than they are.

Sexual Education

Pregnancy and breastfeeding are excellent lessons in human development. During the teenage years, much misinformation is shared on the telephone or in Internet chat rooms, or through rumours. These are big gossip years.

Having a baby in the house can be a wonderful lesson about birth control. While some school sexual education classes require teenagers to lug around 2kg bags of flour for weeks to teach about family planning, teenagers with new babies in their homes should be exempt, as they often have firsthand experience with their new sibling. Learning the responsibilities of infant care firsthand can frighten many teenagers away from early sexual encounters out of fear of pregnancy, or at the very least, can encourage the use of reliable birth control.

Observing a parent breastfeeding an infant teaches important information about the function of the breast in relation to infant nutrition; it also demonstrates bonding in action. Children learn a lot about relationships by watching their parents.

Toolbox Tricks

Teenagers do a lot of journal and diary writing. If you have difficulty communicating verbally with your teenager, write him a letter or send him an e-mail. Children need to know that they are valued and appreciated, and teenagers, like all children, need security and stability, particularly now, when fears of school failure, the future and relationships with the opposite sex are uppermost in their minds. Communicate and spend time with your teenager as best you can.

Teamwork

Pick a good time to discuss with your partner what needs to be done. Agree that your home doesn't need to be spotless – the sooner you get used to some degree of disorganization, the easier it is to be a parent. Children naturally make messes. This is all part of life and part of learning, so don't stress out over little things that aren't really so important in the long run.

Adjusting to life with a new baby is not the time to become fixated on the things that should be done, or should be done differently. You need to concentrate on breastfeeding and caring for your infant. Provide constructive direction to your helpers, and remember that they're still learning, too.

Sometimes it can be hard for mothers to let their partners care for the baby. Remember, your partner doesn't need to interact with your child in the same way you do in order to be a good parent. Each of us has his or her own style, and these styles are all valid as long as they support the safety and healthy development of our children.

Toddlers are big helpers, too. They love to help with housework and copy your behaviour. Give them a mismatched mitten and let them dust the low spots under tables and around the living room. Be sensitive about what they are able to do developmentally and what they are willing to do, based on their mood.

Preschool children often seek ways to assist you before you even ask. They often mimic parents in the roles they play, and have rich imaginations. A well-meaning four-year-old might make you a breakfast of raw carrots with maple syrup to show you that he cares. Young children are helpful at this stage, and are usually willing to fetch nappies and baby wipes; they may even ask to change the nappy themselves. Preschool children can sing and entertain your newborn baby, tell her made-up stories and recite nursery rhymes.

School-age children are a huge help around the house. They usually have their chore lists by now, such as feeding pets, cleaning their rooms or folding their own clothes; you can now slowly increase these chores. Children this age are enthusiastic about changing, holding, rocking and singing lullabies. They can take pictures for the family photo album, offer a bottle of expressed milk, bathe the baby with adult supervision and safety-proof the living room.

Teenagers can offer paid babysitting services, entertainment and increased household responsibility.

The adjustment to new babies is what makes families families. Children learn important life lessons through this experience. Compromise, negotiation, kindness, sharing, trading, humour, cooperation and frustration are all important to survive and be happy in the world.

Family Pets

To prepare your pet for the arrival of your baby, get Dad to bring your infant's unwashed blanket or clothes home on the night before your baby comes home. Allow your pet to have plenty of time exploring her scent.

Before your pet greets your baby, it's important for you to greet him. If you've both been away for a couple of days, your pet will be excited to see you. Greet him first, then while sitting on the sofa, allow him to gently greet your new addition. Introducing your family pet to the new baby should be a slow and gentle process – your pet will learn to recognize and identify your baby through scent, so he will spend a lot of time sniffing (and perhaps sneezing) to commit her smell to memory.

The best pets for small children are those that are gentle, confident, affectionate, loyal, intelligent, patient, sociable, trustworthy and reliable. Even lazy pets are good for babies. Cats are generally good choices.

The best dog breeds for small children include: Labradors, retrievers, bulldogs, boxers, setters, Great Danes, Newfoundlands, Saint Bernards, sheepdogs, collies, beagles and spaniels. Any dogs that are not completely domesticated are poor choices and should be avoided.

As a rule, bigger breeds of dogs do very well with young children, and smaller dogs do not. Some dogs are highly strung, wiry, anxious or emotionally disturbed, or have special needs, and these conditions can affect their behaviour as well as their adaptability to your new baby. Infants develop into curious toddlers, so your pet should be one that children can grow into.

A dog's temperament is inherited but can be changed by both the events in his life and training. It's a unique balance of nature and nurture. Some breeds are friendlier, more intelligent, more tolerant and patient than others; these dogs are also more easily trained.

Never leave a baby or young child unattended with a pet – however trustworthy or well trained – even for a moment. Make sure that you are scrupulous about hygiene.

CHAPTER 19

How Long Should
I Breastfeed?

You are successfully breastfeeding your baby, and everything seems to be going well. Eventually, however, you'll begin to wonder, 'How long should I breastfeed?' Everyone seems to have an opinion on this one: some people will warn you against 'coddling' older infants and toddlers, while others might think it's 'inappropriate' to nurse a child beyond a particular age. In the end, though, the decision is yours.

Physical Limits

How many years can you breastfeed? The short answer is: all of them. Women are generally able to nurse their children as long as they need to. If milk is being taken from the breast, more milk will be produced to take its place. From puberty to death you can produce milk – yes, that long. Menopause is no obstacle.

There's also no physical limit on the age of your nursing child. Although breastmilk is all your baby needs for the first six months of life, older children continue to get immunities and vitamins from your milk for as long as you let them.

Now, just because you can nurse forever, this doesn't mean that you will. Even if you don't actively stop your child from breastfeeding, she will probably stop on her own. If left to the child, breastfeeding usually comes to a natural conclusion by the time she reaches three to four years of age. Of course, you can stop long before then if you decide you want to.

Medical Recommendations

We've established that you could breastfeed your child for years. The real question is 'How long should I breastfeed?', not 'How long can I breastfeed?' There are quite a few recommendations from the medical community and, luckily, they all agree.

- The Royal College of Midwives suggests that all babies should breastfeed exclusively for their first six months.

- The Department of Health also believes that all mothers should nurse exclusively for a minimum of six months.

- The UN's World Health Organization endorses breastfeeding with no other foods for at least the child's first six months of life. In an April 2001 Note to the Press, however, The WHO '… recognizes that some mothers will be unable to, or choose not to, follow this recommendation.'

In short, the medical community says you should breastfeed exclusively for at least your baby's first six months of life. Doctors and researchers recognize the value of breastfeeding with no other supplemental foods for the baby during that first half year. They also recognize the benefits of continued breastfeeding along with other foods until your baby's second birthday and beyond.

tips

Any time spent breastfeeding your child is better than no time at all. The first few weeks of your baby's life are some of the most critical for his health; your breastmilk plays a vital role during this time, and your baby's immune system needs the boost.

So the simple answer is this: you should nurse your baby for at least the first six months, and continue for as long afterwards as both you and your baby want.

Cultural and Historical Issues

Many of the truths we hold as absolute are nothing more than the traditions in which we've been raised. Although some of these traditions are valuable, the ones that interfere with breastfeeding harm children and their families, and modern British culture is not as breastfeeding-friendly as many others around the world are.

In the middle of the last century, breastfeeding became increasingly rare, and with the inception of the NHS and the institutionalization of the birth process, fewer and fewer women chose to breastfeed. Bottle feeding of infant formula was considered more proper and sophisticated by one set of British women, and liberating from traditional roles by another set.

Today, we're lucky. The pendulum of public opinion has swung back in favour of breastfeeding. Accompanying practices such as public nursing, which society once considered 'primitive' or 'unladylike', are becoming increasingly accepted, even unremarkable. At the same time, the increase in popularity that breastfeeding has enjoyed over the past 25 years has raised a new generation that's more supportive of lactation.

Nursing by the Numbers

More and more families are enjoying the benefits of breastfeeding, but the numbers remain lower than health-care professionals would like to see.

In 2000, only 57 per cent of women were still breastfeeding at 1 week, although 71 per cent began to breastfeed at birth. Unfortunately, just 22 per cent were still feeding their babies six months later, and a mere 14 per cent at 9 months old.

The United Kingdom is unusual in this respect, since the average age for complete weaning from the breast worldwide is about four years. Many people feel that the availability of a wide range of nutritious foods makes breastfeeding beyond a year unnecessary, even emotionally harmful, but there is no evidence to support either conclusion. On the contrary, research clearly shows that children benefit from breastmilk until at least their third or fourth birthdays.

Some people will criticize your decision to breastfeed beyond your baby's first few months. Tell the critic your doctor's recommendations. You might even explain the benefits of nursing. To people who say, 'You're still nursing that child?', just smile and tell them, 'Yes. And thanks for noticing!'

Critics of extended breastfeeding believe that it fosters dependence and immaturity. However, growth is a process that can't be rushed – stability, love and security are the foundations of healthy growth, and breastfeeding helps a mother nurture her child's development.

Professional Opinions

Pushing our children to wean before they're ready might actually result in insecurities and bad habits, but most British parents do it anyway. As a result, older toddlers fight to keep their dummies and children entering nursery school still suck their thumbs. The need to suck can't be extinguished by forced weaning.

In the USA, the American Association of Pediatricians puts the blame on a widespread lack of societal support for breastfeeding, pointing to:

· Apathetic and misinformed doctors
· Insufficient breastfeeding education
· Counterproductive hospital policies
· Unnecessary interruption of breastfeeding
· Premature discharge from hospital
· Shortage of routine follow-up care and home health care
· Maternal employment
· Popular media depiction of bottle feeding
· Advertising and promotion of infant formula.

Many researchers would add at least three other items to that list.

Preoccupation with the sexuality of the breast. Western popular culture regards breasts as such inherently sexual organs that their primary function is sometimes threatened. We can't show photos of breastfeeding on billboards for fear of offending someone, so babies with bottles smile out at us from every ad. Even women who breastfeed are often uncomfortable with the idea of nursing a toddler or a preschool child.

Preference for scientific or technological solutions. Bottles and formula strike us as being more scientific than breastfeeding. Western tradition relies heavily on technology, and it's generally paid off for us; however, we've developed an almost religious faith in science and an unhealthy acceptance of infant formula has resulted. We're too quick to assume that a few decades of study can duplicate millions of years of natural selection.

Consumer culture. The Western world can be regarded as a series of nations of consumers, serviced by a huge commercial industry. Breastfeeding just doesn't give us as much to buy as bottle feeding with infant formula does. Corporations push artificial feeding in advertisements and promotions, and manufacturers provide free samples to hospitals and doctors, knowing that an unsure new mother might just decide to use some formula since she has it. After the resulting nipple/teat confusion and decreased milk production, the continued sale of formula is assured.

Women who continue to nurse older children — and there are thousands of them — often keep out of the public eye. No one wants to feel like an outcast because of the way she chooses to care for her child.

Many of us grew up surrounded by baby bottles and infant formula. We used them ourselves and saw them on TV and in magazines. For most Westerners, bottles and formula seem more normal than breastfeeding. However, nature's not a democracy. We can't change what's healthiest for our children by popular practice.

Toddler Nursing

Why nurse a toddler? The benefits of breastfeeding a toddler are the same as they are for younger children.

- Breastmilk continues to be a wonderful source of nutrition, regardless of anything else your child eats.
- Antibodies in your milk continue to protect your toddler, even if he nurses just once a day.
- Breastfeeding comforts children.
- Toddler nursing might be the only snuggling time you get with your busy child while he's awake.
- Breastmilk can be tolerated by unwell children who are unable to stomach other foods.

The more you meet your child's needs, the more independent and confident she will grow. Knowing that you're there for her as she continues to explore gives her the courage to take on a huge, exciting unknown world. Every successful mission will bolster her confidence and increase her sense of independence. Breastfeeding helps.

Styles and Tips

Nursing a toddler presents some unique challenges, but they're usually no problem if you know how to deal with them in advance.

First, how will your child let you know when he wants to nurse? A one-year-old who announces that he wants 'boobies' might be charming around the house, but when he says the same thing in public it can leave you glowing red with embarrassment. This is a problem you can prevent by choosing a good code word for breastfeeding early in your relationship: 'Nurse' is a good one, but anything you like will work.

What do you do with toddler's roaming hands?
Hold your child's hand and kiss his little fingers, or keep a special toy or book nearby that he can hold only while nursing – a textured rattle can sometimes be a good choice. The name of the game is distraction.

If you master the name change, your next hurdle will be explaining that you won't be feeding in public so much anymore. With such a general misunderstanding of toddler nursing in Britain, public feedings can leave you feeling humiliated by the stares and whispers of uninformed strangers. Your child is probably used to nursing whenever he wants – any new restrictions are bound to evoke a tantrum in a headstrong toddler, so be ready for it. This is a good time to begin explaining the difference between 'public' and 'private'. Or you might choose to confidently nurse in public, knowing that you are doing the best for your child.

Toddlers like to move. They've only recently mastered walking, running and climbing, and they love to find new ways to use their bodies. Unfortunately, constant motion and breastfeeding don't go well together. Your little gymnast might decide at some point that nursing would be more fun if he could twist, turn and climb all over you while suckling away. Ouch! Some children can even go from standing to hanging upside down over your shoulder in a single feeding session.

As a child spends less time feeding at his mother's breast, he can spend more time with Dad. This is a great opportunity for early literacy! Dad's lap can be a great refuge to cuddle and read a good book.

If your child's acrobatics are more than you can take, the best solution is to end the breastfeeding session. Don't get angry, but rather announce firmly but gently that nursing time (or whatever you two call it) is a time to lie still. This is the same kind of strategy used to stop nipple biting, and it's usually effective after a very short while.

Your Child's Individual Needs

You are an island of security for your toddler in an unexplored world. Your little adventurer will travel away from you for ever-increasing amounts of time and distance, but he needs to know he can return for protection, comfort and anything else he needs. He's also eager to share what he's experienced with you, and to let you help him understand it.

It's important that you treat your child as an individual. At the same time, pay attention to your own feelings – you're the mother, and you know what's best for your particular child. If you go at the pace that's right for both you and your child, you can continue to enjoy the breastfeeding experience.

Nursing Through Pregnancy

If you're breastfeeding your toddler or older child when you become pregnant, you might be thinking about weaning. However, pregnancy and lactation are more compatible than was once believed, and continued breastfeeding helps an older child feel secure during this time of change.

Obstetricians once routinely advised pregnant women to discontinue breastfeeding for fear of a miscarriage. As we know, nipple stimulation caused by suckling releases oxytocin in your body; this hormone causes a number of things to occur in your body, including milk ejection (letdown) and uterine contractions.

Although oxytocin is released in a pregnant mother's body when she nurses her child, the uterine tissues are less receptive to its effects than they would be if she weren't lactating. Current research seems to indicate that this decreased sensitivity to oxytocin stays strong through the first four months of pregnancy. Even after that time, you can continue to nurse your older child with confidence as long as everything else about your pregnancy is normal.

If you have a history of miscarriages, are diagnosed as 'at risk' for early labour or notice strong contractions while breastfeeding, you should stop nursing your child and contact your doctor immediately. You might be advised to discontinue any nipple stimulation, including sex.

Throughout your pregnancy, you and your toddler will have to accommodate some changes. Beginning at about the fourth month, your breastmilk will decrease in volume and begin to change into the colostrum your newborn needs. Your toddler might or might not take any notice of these changes – some little ones continue right along, nursing as normal, while others will decide that your milk tastes odd and will nurse less frequently.

If you decide to stop breastfeeding, even for a day, it's important for you to find other ways to bond with your toddler. This is also a great opportunity for Dad to spend a little more time with his child. Both parents can read, snuggle and play more with their toddler whenever breastfeeding is interrupted; these other activities will keep him happy and secure in the knowledge that he's not being replaced. With all of the attention the new baby gets, it's common for your older child to feel left out.

Tandem Nursing

Tandem nursing is when you breastfeed two or more children at the same time. It's a great way to keep older children connected with Mum and to teach the value of sharing.

The term 'tandem nursing' is really a misnomer. Most mothers who breastfeed both a newborn and an older child don't do it simultaneously. Usually, the newborn nurses first, and then Mum is available to breastfeed the older child. While common, this approach is not without its drawbacks.

In the first few days of your newborn's life, let him nurse first and nurse as often as he wants. This system of feeding is important to ensure that he receives all the colostrum he needs.

Like serial nursing of twins and triplets, a mother who feeds her toddler after her newborn might feel as if all she does is breastfeed; this can make the process feel less like bonding, and more like an assembly line. Even if you don't mind the arrangement, your toddler might. Depending on how you handled his feedings through your latest pregnancy, your toddler might feel suddenly displaced.

For some mums, simultaneous breastfeeding is the solution. With a child on each breast, nursing takes a lot less time. There's no perceived favourite, and both children stay close to Mum. They might even bond with each other more effectively as they share the satisfaction of nursing. If you find that you don't like it, then try something else. There is no right or wrong answer here – the goal is to find a way to keep all of you happy. Ideally, tandem nursing should be a win-win-win situation.

CHAPTER 20

Infant Nutrition and Introducing Solids

The move to solids is a great time for Dad to get involved in feeding his baby! The first few months of solid food for your baby are good, messy fun. Your baby will love some foods and respond with smiles and squeals. Other foods will make her look at you with expressions of disgust that seem to say, 'What is this horrible stuff you're trying to put in my mouth?'

First Feedings

Infants have an inborn tongue-thrust reflex. They'll push both the spoon and any food on it out of their mouth. This reflex may have evolved to prevent choking, and it continues to be strong until around six months of age. When it comes to infant feeding, most of what goes in will also come out – at one end or the other. Grab your camera, as this will be a perfect photo opportunity: your baby will wear more food than he eats, and you'll want to capture the surprised look on his face when he tries a new taste for the first time. Don't worry that he's not getting enough to eat – more than half his daily calories will continue to be in the form of breastmilk or formula.

WHEN IS BABY READY FOR SOLIDS?

There are some general rules of thumb for assessing whether your baby is prepared for a change of diet. If your baby meets these criteria, he's ready for baby food. Use this checklist to help you assess readiness:

❑ Baby is between four and six months of age.

❑ Baby has doubled his birth weight.

❑ Baby can hold his head upright on his own and turn it from side to side.

❑ Baby can sit up assisted or on his own.

❑ Baby shows an interest in what you're eating and wants some, too.

❑ Baby can communicate when he is full.

❑ Baby is still hungry after a daily total of 1l (32fl oz) of breastmilk or formula.

In time, your baby will learn to swallow solids. Babies swallow differently from a bottle, from a cup and from a straw. They also swallow in a different way with food. A baby has to take food to the roof of his mouth and squash it. Expect your baby to gag or cough the first couple of times; as he develops better tongue control, he will quickly learn to swallow without sputtering.

You can tell that your baby is full if he turns his head away from the food source, closes or clenches his mouth, spits out food or is fretful. These are your cues to end the feeding session.

Follow his first few feedings with breastmilk or formula. As your baby grows, you can offer a cup of water or expressed milk to help wash his food down.

A word about portions: your baby's stomach is the size of his tiny fist, just as your stomach is the size of your grown-up fist. If he eats a tablespoon of cereal followed by a full feeding of breastmilk, he will be satisfied. We often overestimate how much children can eat. Use the 'rule of fist' as your lifelong guide.

The best time to feed will be when you are relaxed and have time to enjoy each other. Babies take a long time to experience food; they savour new flavours and love new textures. Because babies explore the world through sensory play, don't be surprised if mashed potatoes soon become hair gel. It's a messy process, but a necessary one – your baby is learning an important new skill: how to eat!

Supplies

Your baby will need some new supplies as he moves into solid foods – you can finally get to use all those sweet little baby bibs he received as birth gifts! Plastic place mats strategically positioned around the room will catch the leaks from thrown sipping cups and long-distance spills, or you can purchase a large plastic mat to put under the highchair. Even the family pet can help with clearing up.

A plastic or rubber-coated spoon is nice and won't poke your baby's eye out when he tries to use it by himself. You might consider letting him play with the spoon for a few days before starting solids so that he can become familiar with it. Chewing on a coated spoon also helps when your baby's gums are sensitive from teething. A divided plastic dish with high sides is perfect for feeding several different foods at one time, such as fruits, vegetables and cereal; if the plate has suction cups to stick it to the highchair tray, all the better.

Food Allergies

Although food allergies are rare, they do occur. The foods most likely to cause allergies include: peanut products, strawberries, milk products, citrus fruits, tomatoes, egg whites, fish, spinach and wheat. Wait until your baby is at least a year old before sharing these foods with her.

Keep a notebook to record your baby's reactions to new foods. If your baby experiences rash, excessive phlegm, coughing, wheezing, watery eyes, diarrhoea, vomiting, hives or any respiratory ailment after the introduction of a new food, contact your doctor.

Foods to Avoid

Some everyday foods are not suitable for infants:

Nuts – Avoid giving whole nuts to children under five years old because of the risk of choking.

Salt – Never add salt to your baby's food, as his digestive system cannot cope with higher salt levels than those found naturally in foods.

Sugar – Do not add sugar to any of your baby's food, as high consumption of sugar causes tooth decay and will also encourage your child to develop a sweet tooth.

Honey – As well as being a very rich source of sugar, honey can contain spores that are very dangerous for babies. Do not give honey to children under one year old.

In addition, if you have a family history of food allergy, speak to your doctor or health visitor before giving the following to your baby:

Dairy products
Eggs
Citrus fruit (and juices)
Shellfish
Wheat and wheat-based products – including rusks
Any nuts or seeds – including peanut butter.

Food Schedules

Foods should be introduced slowly and one at a time. Allow at least three days between introductions so you can identify potential problems. If you have a family history of food allergies, remember to pay special attention to your baby's reactions to new foods.

Cereals

Because babies' digestive systems are still immature, they need foods that are easily absorbed. Infant cereals should be the first foods following breastmilk or formula that baby will experience.

Start with a box of dry rice cereal. Boxes are better bargains than jars, and dry cereals allow you to add human milk or formula. Rice also has the fewest allergy-related reactions. Wait at least a week between introducing new cereals: rice should be followed by oatmeal, then barley. Wheat and mixed cereals can cause allergic reactions in infants younger than one year of age, so it's better to wait before introducing these.

Juice

Juice can be introduced at around six to eight months of age. Start with 100 per cent grape juice, as this is easiest to digest – apple and pear juices, although milder than other fruit juices, contain sorbital, a natural fruit sugar our intestines cannot absorb: it ferments in the intestines and causes stomach aches and diarrhoea. Grape juice does not contain sorbital. Acidic juices, such as cranberry, orange and grapefruit, should be delayed until after your baby's first birthday.

In the case of juice, more is not better, as it can cause rapid tooth decay because of its high sugar content. It's important that juice is fed only in a cup, not a bottle, and that a regular toothbrushing routine is established. Juice can also cause obesity and digestive problems, so its use should be limited.

Choose only 100 per cent fruit juices. Some doctors recommend that juice be diluted to half-strength, but government sources do not. Avoid cans or bottles labelled 'juice drink': these have only a small amount of juice added, and the first ingredient listed – all too often, sugar – is the main ingredient. Learning to read labels now will help you to make healthy choices as your child grows.

From six to 12 months of age, only 125ml (4fl oz) of juice is recommended per day. You can serve small amounts throughout the day or offer one full cup at a sitting. Juice will curb your baby's appetite, so offer it as a snack between meals. As baby gets older, whole unprocessed fruits are a better choice than juice.

Vegetables

Join the 'vegetables first' crowd. Babies already have a preference for sweet things, so fruits will be readily accepted. Some vegetables, on the other hand, might take some getting used to, and your baby might refuse to eat vegetables if fruits are introduced first.

Baby vegetables come pureed or strained. They have the consistency of apple sauce, but not necessarily the texture. Some manufacturers add modified tapioca food starch as a filler to smooth the texture, but this has little or no nutritional value.

Vegetables can be introduced at around six months of age. One to two tablespoons per day is all your baby needs for the next three months. A yellow vegetable at lunch and a green vegetable with dinner will provide a balanced and nutritious diet for your baby.

 Spinach, beetroot and broccoli cause wind and should be avoided until after 12 months of age. They are also high in naturally occurring nitrates, which reduce your baby's ability to transport oxygen through his blood. Use these foods moderately.

Add one new vegetable per week, and watch out for reactions such as allergies or nappy rash.

Fruits

Fruits will be enthusiastically explored and accepted by your baby. Fruits without added sugars are best, so mash peaches tinned in their own juice or grate a fresh pear. As with vegetables, one to two tablespoons of fruit per day is all a baby needs for healthy development. Add one new fruit per week, and again watch for signs of allergic reaction.

There are a few precautions you need to take when serving fruits to your baby: citrus fruits should be avoided until after your baby's first birthday; dried fruits are sticky and can cause cavities; apple slices, as well as other raw fruits and vegetables, can be a choking hazard. When your baby is old enough to tolerate oranges and tangerines, remember to remove the pips.

Meats

Meats are generally introduced at around nine months of age, and are important sources of iron and protein. Instead of buying potted meats, you can simply save a few tablespoons of unseasoned meat you've cooked for supper and mash it for your baby. Making your own ground chicken, pork, beef or turkey costs less than commercially prepared foods. Serve meats cooked through and warm but not hot.

Eggs should be cooked and egg whites should be removed, as they are an allergen. Hard-boil an egg and serve the mashed yolk. If your baby develops an allergy to eggs before his first birthday, tell your GP.

Breastmilk and Bottles

Some mothers nurse before offering solids to take the edge off baby's appetite, while others wait to nurse until afterwards. Try both ways. You know your baby best and whatever you choose will be right for him.

It's important to continue breastfeeding as your baby learns to eat solid food. When infants are six months of age or younger, solids are not a substitute for breastmilk – they are a supplement to breastfeeding. Your milk contains the nutrients your baby needs, and because he's still getting the majority of his calories through your milk, nursing should be continued.

However, older babies tend to breastfeed less and take fewer bottles as they eat more and more solids. This is often the time when most babies decide to self-wean. Weaning is accelerated by introducing new foods to an infant's diet.

RECOMMENDED DAILY ALLOWANCE OF FOOD FOR INFANTS UNDER ONE YEAR OF AGE

AGE	FOOD	SERVINGS	AMOUNT PER SERVING
0–4 months	Breastmilk	8–12	
	Formula	4–8	up to 1l (32fl oz)
4–6 months	Breastmilk	6–8	
	Formula	4–8	up to 1l (32fl oz)
	Cereal	2	1–2 tablespoons
6–9 months	Breastmilk	5–7	
	Formula	4	up to 1l (32fl oz)
	Cereal	2	2–4 tablespoons
	Vegetables	2	2 tablespoons
	Fruits	2	2 tablespoons
	Juice	1	60–125ml (2–4fl oz)
9–12 months	Breastmilk	4–5	
	Formula	4	up to 1l (32fl oz)
	Cereal	2	3–4 tablespoons
	Vegetables	2	3–4 tablespoons
	Fruits	2	3–4 tablespoons
	Juice	1	60–125ml (2–4fl oz)
	Bread	2	1/2 slice
	Crackers		1–2
	Meats	2	3–4 tablespoons

Safe Handling and Storage of Baby Foods

You were careful to ensure clean hands and breasts when you started nursing. Cleanliness is even more important now, as you can't always know where food has been or what it's been exposed to.

It's also important to serve baby foods from a dish, not straight from the jar. For smaller infants, you can measure the appropriate amounts in divided containers. Throw away any uneaten food from the dish: bacteria from baby's mouth will contaminate the food and continue to grow, and that could make your baby ill.

BABY FOOD STORAGE: HOMEMADE OR OPENED JARS		
FOOD	REFRIGERATOR	FREEZER
Fruits	2–3 days	6–8 months
Vegetables	2–3 days	6–8 months
Meats	1 day	1–2 months
Eggs	1 day	1–2 months
Mixed foods	1–2 days	1–2 months

Finger Foods

At around seven to nine months, offer your child finger foods. Bite-size pieces of unsalted crackers, toast (avoid wholemeal), and unsweetened pieces of cereals are great foods for little mouths and hands. Baby is developing an ability to draw his thumb and fingers together to pick up small items (including the fluff under your sofa) and bring them to his mouth. His saliva will quickly transform crackers to mush, but whole rusks or broken bits of teething biscuits can make him choke. Keep an eye on all finger foods – babies will sometimes swallow without chewing, so caution is recommended.

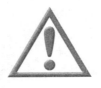

The following foods are extremely chokeable and should be avoided until after your baby's first birthday: popcorn, marshmallows, nuts (including peanuts), sweets, pretzels, raw vegetables, grapes, hot dogs and peanut butter. Babies put almost everything in their mouth. Now is the time to enrol in an infant first aid and CPR class.

Dairy products such as cottage or string cheeses and frozen yogurt can be introduced around your baby's first birthday, as can whole pasteurized milk. At this age, babies need less than 1l (32fl oz) of milk per day. Make sure to use whole milk, not semi-skimmed, skimmed or chocolate milk. The fat in whole milk is important for brain development. Offer milk in a cup but not in a bottle, which can now be used for water at bedtime. Water will often help your toddler lose interest in the bottle, making it easier to let go.

Brushing Teeth

You can begin to clean an infant's gums even before the eruption of her first tooth; a small piece of moist gauze is sufficient. After the first tooth comes through, at around five to six months of age, you can offer a cool, damp flannel to chew on between and after meals.

After your baby's first birthday, introduce a toddler toothbrush, which can be purchased at any chemist or pharmacy. These toothbrushes are smaller than child-sized brushes and have fewer bristles. Use only water to clean teeth, since toddlers will often swallow toothpaste.

Visit a dentist between the ages of two and three. She will tell you when to begin flossing and will provide additional dental education.

Most importantly, remember to practise good dental hygiene and your baby will follow your lead.

CHAPTER 21

Employment, Child Care and Breastfeeding

Breastfeeding when you return to work can be a challenge: it requires a lot of commitment and determination to maintain your milk supply and to stand up for yourself and your baby. You need the support of all the players on your team – the assistance of the right child care provider, a supportive employer and a breastfeeding-friendly workplace can help to ensure your continued success.

Finding Breastfeeding-Friendly Day Care

The search for day care often begins before your baby is even born. The best places have lengthy waiting lists, and rightly so – in the day care business, you often get what you pay for.

It's especially important to find a provider who shares your parenting philosophies. Make a list of key issues that are important to you and discuss them with each potential caregiver. Be sure to ask questions about their policies and procedures on breastfeeding and the handling and storage of breastmilk. There are several types of day care environments to consider, from commercial care centres to private, in-home care. Only you know what's best for your baby.

Nurseries

Most nurseries are licensed facilities that meet regulated national health and safety standards; officials maintain quality through random observations and inspections. Consider the following pros and cons as you list your priorities and do your research.

ADVANTAGES VERSUS DISADVANTAGES OF NURSERIES	
ADVANTAGES	**DISADVANTAGES**
They are often licensed or registered.	Children are often exposed to illness from other babies.
Care is monitored by other staff and the director.	Noisy, busy environments can overstimulate babies.
Staff are often certified in CPR and first aid.	Having several providers can be confusing to your infant.
Staff often have childcare qualifications or receive specialized training in child development.	Hours usually range from 9:00 AM to 5.00 or 6:00 PM, without flexibility.
Educational programmes are offered.	Staff turnover may be high.
There are opportunities for babies to interact and socialize.	Some nurseries are expensive.
When staff become ill, other providers can fill in.	

Before you make a decision about a nursery, ask the care providers and staff these questions:

- Is the nursery registered?
- What is the policy on the handling and storage of breastmilk?

· Is there a place I can nurse my baby after work or during breaks?
· What are your hours of opening?
· What is the cost?
· Are activities structured or child-driven?
· How many children are cared for by each member of staff?
· Are staff trained in CPR and first aid?
· Is there clear communication between the nursery and parents in the form of meetings, newsletters or parent groups?
· What are your policies on discipline, emergencies, bad weather, dispensing medications and illness?
· Will I be charged if my infant is ill and absent from the nursery?

As you go around the nursery, pay special attention to the atmosphere and activities. Are the rooms and toys clean and inviting? Are the children engaged in developmentally appropriate activities? Do the children seem happy? Are crying babies attended and soothed? Is the environment clean and safe for young children?

Don't be shy! Ask for references from other parents with infants the same age as your baby. Phone them and ask them to describe the quality of care their babies receive in the nursery, as well as the pros and cons of placing children in this nursery's care. When you enroll, ask for copies of all policies and procedures, and get a copy of your contract. Day care is a business deal. Enter into it carefully.

Registered Childminders

Many parents today choose a childminder to provide day care. Family day care is offered in the home of the childminder, who usually has up to six children of varying ages in her care. Many new parents like the intimacy of this kind of day care.

By law, childminders must be registered with your local authority; in addition to personal recommendation or advertisements, you can find a childminder by phoning your local authority, who will have a list that tells you where your nearest childminder is to be found.

ADVANTAGES VERSUS DISADVANTAGES OF CHILDMINDERS

ADVANTAGES	DISADVANTAGES
Child care occurs in a natural, home setting.	Alternative care may be unavailable if the provider is sick or on holiday.
Childminders are often inexpensive.	They are harder to monitor for quality of care.
Mixed-age groups allow children interaction through a variety of socialization experiences.	Children may be exposed to illness.
One consistent caregiver forms a relationship with your infant.	
Some providers offer flexible weekend and evening hours.	
Registered with the local authority.	

When considering the options of a childminder, you should be just as clear in your expectations and priorities as you would at any other 'commercial' facility. Exercise your right to ask the childminder these questions:

- Is your home licensed or registered?
- What is your policy on the handling and storage of breastmilk?
- Is space available to breastfeed my baby?
- How many children are in your care?
- Do you have back-up support during family illness or holidays?
- Do you transport children in an insured vehicle? Do you have a valid driver's licence?
- Are car seats available?
- Are you trained in CPR and first aid?
- What are your policies on discipline, emergencies, bad weather, dispensing medications and ill children?
- Can my baby still attend if he is ill?
- Is there still a charge if my infant is absent from day care?
- What are your hours of operation? Do you offer flexible hours?
- What is the cost?

Interview likely candidates more than once, and bring your baby to at least one of the interviews to observe his interaction with the childminder and the childminder's ease with your infant. You may also want to get a feeling about your infant's ease with another childminder. Many infants need time to get used to someone else, but at least you'll get a preview of what you can expect.

When is the best time to visit a child care facility?
Schedule a tour of any childminder's premises in the early morning or late afternoon. Most babies take a nap mid-morning or after lunch, and you want to observe activity and interaction between the childminder and the children in her care.

Make a point of discussing parenting philosophies regarding such topics as breastfeeding, discipline, crying babies, colic, bonding, dummy use, feeding styles and potty learning with your intended provider. If the childminder disagrees with your philosophies, find out whether she is willing to accept and follow your preferences over her own.

In-Home Day Care

In-home care is an option that allows others to provide care for your baby in his own natural environment, his home. This kind of care can be expensive, and those with the financial resources often employ live-in nannies. A more cost-effective option for most would be to employ a friend or family member.

If possible, arrange to be at home with the provider for the first week, but keep a low profile. Your baby and the provider will need some time to get used to being with and around each other, while you'll need to get used to having a stranger care for your child in your own home.

ADVANTAGES VERSUS DISADVANTAGES OF IN-HOME CARE

ADVANTAGES	DISADVANTAGES
Your baby remains in familiar surroundings with all supplies needed for his care.	It's difficult to monitor the quality of care your infant receives.
Your baby receives consistency of care and full attention from one individual who will develop a relationship with him.	It's difficult to find someone outside the family who can place the same investment in your child as you do.
Flexible hours may include evenings and weekends.	Alternative care if your in-home caregiver is ill may be difficult to find.
Your baby is not exposed to illness from other children.	It's a high-stress job and has high turnover rates (about 90 per cent annually).
Parents do not have to pack up little ones on cold mornings and transport them to day care.	It's expensive.
If a parent must travel, in-home care can provide around-the-clock supervision.	It can be isolating, with little peer-group interaction for your growing baby.

Because you are dealing with an individual – a free agent, of sorts – you need to ask different questions and do additional and thorough research. Ask all candidates for an in-home care position these questions:

· What previous experience do you have with newborn care?
· What are the costs/fees involved?
· What special arrangements will you require (benefits, private room, evenings and weekends free)?
· Do you smoke, drink or use drugs?
· Do you have transport and a valid driver's licence, and are you insured?
· Do you have any health concerns that might interfere with the job?
· Can you work flexible hours?
· Are there other children (her own) in your care?
· Can you provide full-time care, if needed?
· Why did you leave your last job?
· Have you ever been charged with a crime?

Ask for references and contact them. Every one of them. Ask if they would hire this person again. Were they pleased with the quality of care? Were there any concerns of which you should be aware?

Listen to your intuition when making a final decision. If something just doesn't seem right, you can either interview a third time or find another provider. You want to make the best decision based on all available information.

Breastfeeding and Day Care

Ask your provider not to feed your baby within an hour of when you plan to arrive. If your baby is hungry, ask your provider to feed her just enough to take the edge off of her appetite. That means you'll need to have extra breastmilk available at day care, especially if your baby receives breastmilk exclusively – formula supplements take longer to digest, and your baby might not be hungry when you arrive to nurse her.

If you've established a sound breastfeeding routine and you think your baby is ready for a dummy, you can ask your provider to offer your baby her 'plug' throughout the day. This will help meet her need to suck and may stave off hunger until you arrive.

Many babies suffer from nipple/teat confusion when they are not used to supplements or expressed milk in a bottle. The milk smells like their mother's, but the containers and teats are different. Some babies adamantly refuse the bottle: they will let go of the teat, thrash their heads, reattach, become frustrated and cry.

Practise using a bottle for a few feedings before the first day of day care. Babies can also be cup fed or spoon fed, or offered milk in a feeding syringe. Older infants can use a straw or sipping cup. Work closely with your provider to develop a feeding system that works for everyone.

Other causes for feeding difficulties at day care include a change of environment, noise levels, different smells and constant activity. Talk to your child care provider about your baby's feeding schedules. Remember that your baby will eat when he's hungry and will stop when he's full.

Returning to Work

Almost half of the UK work force is female. Because of this, special considerations are now being given to make breastfeeding and employment more compatible.

Returning to work should be a gradual process. Talk to your employer before you start maternity leave. Discuss the possibility of returning at part-time status or for half-days for the first few weeks back. Ask if you can return on a Thursday or Friday, creating a long transitional weekend to get mentally prepared and back on track. Other options to consider include job sharing, working from home or flexible scheduling. Some small businesses might allow your young, non-mobile infant to come to work with you. Research the policies or benefits that are offered for breastfeeding women.

Breastfeeding-Friendly Employment Environments

Being family-friendly is good business and good for business! What makes a company family-friendly? Consider companies that:

· Offer paid parental leave or give options to take longer unpaid parental leaves without the threat of job loss
· Offer on-site child care or work with community child care providers
· Provide nursing breaks for breastfeeding mums (two 30-minute breaks, plus lunch) and provide separate rooms where mothers can express and store their milk.

While this may sound expensive for an employer, it's really to the company's advantage. Offering these kinds of benefits decreases employee absenteeism and turnover. Maintaining qualified personnel by offering lactation rooms returns a huge payoff. Babies who are breastfed fall ill less often, so parents have fewer sick days. Employees feel supported and valued: they have higher morale and productivity, enhanced loyalty to their company and lower insurance claims. This action also improves the company's position and status in the community.

Maintaining Your Milk Supply

Begin to stockpile your milk for at least a week before returning to work. Express on the weekends and throughout the day, just as you would after your baby nurses.

As you pump milk at work, you might notice a decrease in production during the first week. This is normal. You'll continue to produce an abundant supply if you follow a regular pumping schedule and nurse your baby frequently when you return home. She can empty the breast more efficiently that any breast pump can.

fact

You may encounter colleagues who seem resentful of the time you are spending expressing your milk, especially if they have to assume your responsibilities while you are away from your desk. Don't take this to heart. Show your appreciation to colleagues by sending them a thank-you note from your baby.

Nurse early in the morning, then again before you leave for work: your milk supply is most abundant in the mornings when you have higher levels of prolactin. Express milk throughout the day, and nurse your baby again when you pick him up from day care. Many child care providers offer a quiet space to nurse your baby and can also have your baby awake and ready to nurse when you arrive if you phone in advance.

Breastfeeding at Work

If you are planning to return to work while breastfeeding, it's a good idea to discuss your needs with your employer before you actually start work again. It may help to write down your position in a letter, explaining how you plan to combine working with expressing, plus a letter from your GP or health visitor explaining the benefits of continued breastfeeding. It is worth telling your employer that maternal absences from work are fewer when the baby is breastfed than when she is fed formula. Explain what you will need to express at work. You will need access to a fridge so that you can store the milk safely, and you should also have access to an electric socket. Ask your employer if they have a written breastfeeding policy. By law you are entitled to some protection, but it is important to notify your employer in writing that you are breastfeeding:

Your employer must ensure your working environment is safe and that you do not come into contact with any chemicals or other substances that might adversely affect your milk.

Your employer must provide somewhere suitable for you to express – and this is not the ladies' toilet. Ask if there is an unused office or other space that you could make comfortable. Make sure the space is clean. Remember you will have to take all your equipment to the office – including something to sterilize your feeding equipment – so you will need an adequate space to store whatever you need. You are entitled to a space with a lockable door.

If you work in the public sector you are covered by the European Pregnant Worker's Directive. This states that your employer must also ensure that your working hours and conditions allow you to continue breastfeeding for as long as you like.

According to the International Labour Organization's Maternity Protection Convention, breastfeeding women should be entitled to at least one break a day to express milk, and that there should be no drop in pay or addition to working hours as a result.

For more information about breastfeeding at work, contact the Maternity Alliance (0207 588 8582).

Staying at Home

Research findings conclude that returning to work is correlated with decreased breastfeeding rates, but making the decision not to return to work can be difficult. Most women believe they must work for financial reasons. However, many have found that staying at home with their child is less of a financial sacrifice than they feared. The often-overlooked truth of the matter is that most families' second incomes are far less profitable than they think. We see the figure on our wage slips, but don't always fully consider how much is spent in related costs.

One study by the US Department of Labor found that about 80 per cent of a working mother's income is absorbed by job-related expenses. It's not even unusual for couples to discover that their second income is entirely consumed by work-related expenses.

Here are a few factors to consider in making a decision about returning to work or staying home.

Career paths. Many women have invested a great deal of time and effort into their careers and enjoy working too much to consider staying at home. You might decide that your career goals would be compromised by an interruption. Your needs and desires must always be an important consideration.

Clothing and travelling expenses. The cost of commuting can be substantial, whether you drive or take the bus or train. For some urban families, one vehicle would be enough were it not for the second job. Car maintenance, parking, petrol and services all add up. Then there's the cost of maintaining a professional wardrobe: you'll still need smart clothes for some occasions, but not as many, and they'll last longer.

Cost of day care. Day care can be expensive. You can expect to pay at least £400–600 per month for infant care, depending on what type you choose. As discussed earlier, childminders are the least expensive, and in-home care is the most expensive. If you have more than one child, expenses could double.

Food expenses at work versus home. Unless you're the kind of person who takes in an inexpensive lunch every day, workday food expenses can really put a dent in your purse. The average homemade lunch costs less than £1, while the very cheapest fast-food meal is more than twice that. That's over £480 per year, not counting trips to the vending machine for snacks. The other, often hidden, food expense to consider is the cost of getting a takeaway at night because everyone is too tired or impatient to prepare a meal.

Intellectual stimulation and camaraderie. Staying at home can be very isolating and even boring at times. Your baby is always happy to interact with you, but sometimes you'll miss adult conversation and the friendly camaraderie of your fellow employees. Many stay-at-home parents start playgroups, write newsletters, take up hobbies and volunteer at schools to combat feelings of isolation.

Self-esteem and social status. Many people define themselves in terms of what they do, and losing that role can leave some parents feeling depressed or diminished. There's a real lack of appreciation in the world for the hard work, skill and ingenuity of stay-at-home parents.

Time. Time is money, so they say. Much of the expense of the dual-income lifestyle originates in lost time. You don't have time to paint the living room, so you employ a painter. You don't have time to cook, so you get takeaways. You don't have time to shop for the best prices, so you buy whatever you can get quickly. Convenience is the hot new benefit offered in today's marketplace, and it costs money. Moderately careful stay-at-home parents can sometimes save more than they would earn at a job, simply by investing their time wisely.

If you find that your job is less profitable than you thought, maybe it's time to consider becoming a full-time parent for a while. On the other hand, if you're unable to stay at home, there are other solutions. You could jobshare, work part-time or run your business out of a home office.

JOB-RELATED EXPENSES WORKSHEET

Taxes
(Taken from your salary and possibly your partner's)   £ _____

Work clothing   £ _____
(Purchase price, wear, dry cleaning)

Transport   £ _____
(Car payment, parking, petrol, insurance)

Eating out/snacks   £ _____
(List only the difference over home cooking)

Day care   £ _____

Office gifts
   (Birthdays, funeral flowers, etc.)   £ _____

Convenience services   £ _____
   (Things you could do if you had time)

Total expenses: £ _____

Gross income: £ _____

Value of your job (Income – expenses):   £ _____

Stay-at-Home Dads

More and more fathers are moving away from employment outside the home to full-time fathering and housekeeping while Mum goes off to work. It's an arrangement that benefits the entire family: mothers can continue on their career paths uninterrupted, knowing that their children are being cared for by someone who loves them, and fathers can enjoy the special parent–child relationship that usually belongs to Mum.

65 per cent of stay-at-home fathers surveyed in the USA, and 78 per cent of their partners, chose their arrangement because they wanted their child to be raised by a parent. The secondary reason in many of the studied cases was financial. The mothers made more money, a situation that's no longer unusual.

Rather than having a simple reversal of household roles, families with stay-at-home dads tend to be more balanced. Parental power and responsibilities are more evenly divided than in more traditional family arrangements.

Couples considering this move need to consider all the factors listed earlier, paying special attention to the social and emotional criteria. There aren't very many traditional role models for stay-at-home fathers, and studies show that the isolation of staying at home and the loss of self-esteem and status from leaving their jobs still hits men harder than it hits women.

However, staying at home with your child is a richly rewarding experience that few people of either gender would fail to appreciate. Fortunately for men, it's an opportunity that's becoming more common every day.

CHAPTER 22

Weaning

When to wean depends on both you and your baby. Some babies lose interest in nursing once solids are offered or the cup is introduced, others nurse happily until they become mobile and begin to move towards independence, while still others are content to nurse throughout their preschool years. The methods you use differ depending on who's initiating the process.

Nursing Strike versus Weaning

Sometimes, completely out of the blue, a baby decides he doesn't want to nurse. He'll purse his lips, refuse the breast and cry. This may last for one feeding or for several days. It can be hard to tell if your baby is ill, self-weaning or holding a nursing strike.

Many mums mistake a nursing strike for self-weaning and give up breastfeeding long before their babies are ready. Babies who self-wean usually lose interest gradually over a period of time or are more distractible at the breast; in contrast, most nursing strikes happen suddenly and while babies are still very young.

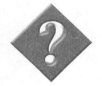

What can cause a nursing strike?
Babies choose not to nurse for a variety of reasons; teething can be a big factor; swallowing and jaw movement might be painful for your baby if he's suffering from an earache, mouth injury or sore throat; or maybe your baby senses stress or anxiety – even changes such as a new deodorant or perfume can cause confusion.

The solution? If at first you don't succeed, try, try, try again. Offer the breast when your baby is sleepy, as he is less likely to fight it when he's tired. Offer to nurse again as your baby wakes – the quiet-alert state is best. Some suggest that simply changing feeding positions or nursing while walking helps.

If your baby still refuses to nurse, express your milk and offer it in an infant feeding cup, a spoon, a syringe, an eyedropper or a sipping cup.

Your milk supply is regulated by your baby's demand, and when your baby refuses to nurse, your body slows production. Nursing strikes usually don't exceed beyond four days, but by that time, your milk supply could decrease. To maintain your supply, express milk manually or with a breast pump as often as your baby would normally nurse.

After 24 hours of baby's refusal of the breast, it's time to call your GP or health visitor, as your baby may need a check-up to rule out health conditions such as thrush or ear infection.

Remember: your baby is not rejecting you; he is temporarily rejecting the breast. In a short while, the cause of the strike will resolve and you'll resume your breastfeeding relationship.

Special Situations: Sudden Weaning

Abrupt weaning can be difficult and uncomfortable for both mother and baby. It can lead to engorgement and breast infections, as well as feelings of depression and loss for Mum. It can also lead to nipple/teat confusion if your baby is transitioned to a bottle for the first time.

Teething and the Breast

Teething can hurt – especially when teeth are bursting out like popcorn. The process can disrupt the breastfeeding relationship if it's simply too painful for your baby to nurse. Your baby may refuse the breast, or she may bite you to help work her teeth through. The initial shock and pain may cause you to reflexively shout, which will, in turn, scare your baby and may cause her to refuse the breast the next time it's offered.

Sudden weaning can cause clogged ducts or breast infection. See your GP or health visitor if you experience fever, chills, heat in your breast or flu-like symptoms. You may need to be treated with antibiotics.

If you're aware of the signs of teething, you can be on guard against biting before it happens. Signs of teething include:

- Biting everything in sight, from spoons and sipping cup lids to you and unsuspecting playmates
- Nappy rash from diarrhoea caused by the acids in excess saliva
- Dribbling
- Rash or chapped chin
- Tearfulness

Teething does not have to be a reason to wean, although many parents use this event as a time to move babies to the bottle.

The Emotional Rollercoaster

As prolactin levels decrease, you may begin to experience a temporary bout of baby blues, characterized by feelings of sadness, tearfulness, decrease in appetite, confusion, insomnia and mood swings. You may have put off this postnatal phenomenon because you made the decision to breastfeed – but with sudden weaning you may begin to experience these symptoms for the first time.

These feelings will pass as your hormones balance themselves again, but it's important to eat well, exercise, take time for yourself and find a supportive person to talk to.

Stopping Your Milk Production

Stopping breastfeeding in one sudden go is usually an unnecessary process. Ideally, weaning is a gradual process – when you wean suddenly, the results can be painful.

Engorgement caused by rapid weaning can leave you with full, painful breasts. When this happens, express just enough milk to make yourself comfortable, but remember that milk is made by supply and demand. When you express milk, it will be replaced with more. Milk remaining in the breast signals your body that you have more milk than you're using, and will slow production.

There are several other methods you can use to decrease milk production and the pain of engorgement.

Cabbage Leaves

Earlier, you learned that cool cabbage leaves tucked into your bra can relieve engorgement. You also learned not to use them for too long or too often because they slow milk production. Now your goal is to slow production, so feel free to use them as much as you need to.

Leaves should be changed when they begin to wilt. During weaning, cabbage leaves can be worn around the clock.

Oestrogen

Oestrogen, as discussed earlier, is a hormone that reduces milk production. Some birth control pills contain high levels of oestrogen, which will decrease your milk supply. However, many birth control pills on the market today are oestrogen-free. Talk to your doctor before asking for a prescription.

Transitioning Baby: Gradual Weaning

Gradual weaning begins with a plan. Look at a calendar to put this in perspective. You'll need six to eight weeks for a comfortable transition, and the more time you take, the less traumatic it will be for both you and your child.

Gradual weaning will help you maintain a healthy hormonal balance. Because your hormone levels will decrease more slowly in time, you'll feel fewer symptoms of the baby blues. The key to keeping mood swings in check is proceeding slowly.

A gradual transition will also keep lactation in balance. Mothers who wean slowly don't experience engorgement. Your weaning infant or toddler will help your body produce just the right amount of milk.

Reduced Feedings

When is your baby least interested in nursing? Mid-morning? Early evening? Those will be the first feedings to eliminate, but only one at a time. If you decide to wean in two months, work out which sessions to eliminate, as well as new activities or foods to substitute.

Keep an eye on toddlers who are slow to accept change: weaning can be scary and stressful for them. Avoid emotional battles over the breast. Slow-to-transition children need more time to accept change. Flexibility is important!

Decrease your nursing schedule by one session every five days. For example, eliminate mid-morning nursing, and after five days, begin to eliminate early-evening sessions. Bedtimes and naptimes will be the last to go, because babies often suck for comfort on these occasions. Nighttime feedings are usually the most difficult to give up. Patience and consistency are key; inconsistency will only delay the process.

Offer the breast less frequently and for shorter amounts of time. A delayed nursing session might even make a busy toddler forget. Don't refuse your child the breast, but don't offer it frequently.

Change Routines

When it's time to eliminate that final nursing session of the day, rethink the bedtime routine. Give your baby a bath, read a story, drink a cup of water, brush her teeth, put on a lullaby tape, give a brief massage, kiss and say goodnight. If you've weaned to the bottle, let Dad offer a bottle of water and initiate the bedtime routine.

Your partner can also spend time alone with your weaning baby: an afternoon out together, a walk around the block or cuddling during storytime will distract a busy toddler from wanting the breast.

It's often helpful to eliminate the feeding cues that remind your baby that it's time to nurse: sit on the sofa instead of the chair; face baby forwards in the sling rather than towards your breast.

If your baby is six months of age, offer her a sipping cup with expressed breastmilk, 100 per cent grape juice or water. A new taste, along with the novelty of the cup, will appeal to her. You can also replace a nursing session with the introduction of a new solid food. But remember to try new foods one at a time, and watch for signs of allergy.

Offer the cup following a feeding of solids and expect a mess. Remember: babies are moist and they learn through their senses. Wet is good to a baby – and slidy, squishy, squirmy wet is even better.

What's the best way to get your baby used to a cup?
Begin to introduce the cup at between six and nine months of age. Babies develop the ability to move objects from hand to hand in the middle of their bodies (midline) at around six months. By nine months, this skill is well mastered and babies are ready to manipulate cups with lids.

Expect the cup to become a new toy for your baby. He'll throw it and expect you to pick it up (over and over and over again). This game is not played to frustrate you, nor is it a sign of sipping cup palsy. Your baby is learning cause and effect ('If I throw it, you'll pick it up... every time!') and object permanence (out of sight is not out of mind). Both these concepts are important for normal development, and you've just provided the right age-appropriate toy to teach them.

Gradual Weaning by Age

Your weaning plan should take into account your child's age and developmental abilities. A child who is moving towards independence is more distractible than a child who has a much more predictable routine. Think about the ages and stages of your child when developing your weaning plan.

0–6 months: Wean from the breast to a bottle. Babies still have a need to suck. To avoid battles, offer the bottle to your baby when he is neither too tired nor too hungry. Babies at this age will often experience nipple/teat confusion. Vary feeding positions, try different bottle teats, and get someone else to offer the bottle if he rejects it from you.

6–12 months: You can gradually replace breastfeeding sessions with solid foods and the introduction of the cup. Offer the cup more frequently. A dummy can meet your baby's need to suck. Infants at this age are more distractible, so a change in routine can help them make the change from the breast more easily.

12–24 months: Your toddler is moving towards independence and is mastering self-help skills. Toddlers at this age can now successfully manipulate a cup. Use the cup more frequently and begin to offer water in the bottle, if your child is using one. Your toddler is now eating table foods and has a varied diet. He sleeps through the night and doesn't rely on late-night feedings. This is the ideal age to introduce transitional objects for security (teddy bears and blankets) and to wean from the bottle. Teach your baby other ways to comfort himself.

24–36 months: At this age, toddlers are active, curious and always on the go. You can substitute activities, such as trips to the park or playground, in place of nursing. A change in routine will help eliminate nursing cues. Use a cup during cuddle times. Children love to listen to stories and make up their own. Replace nursing sessions with lap time in a different chair.

36 months and over: Children at this age nurse for emotional closeness. They prefer to play but still need to feel the safety of their parents. Invite friends over to play more frequently. Get Dad to offer days out with your preschool child as a change in routine.

If you have concerns with your baby's development with respect to his age, discuss your weaning options or plan with your GP or health visitor. Again, you know your child best and are the most qualified judge of what methods will work for you and your family.

Weaning from Breast to Bottle

Introduction to the bottle should be a gradual process. Bottle teats aren't like human nipples, and infants suck differently from breast to bottle to cup. The teat flow from a bottle releases milk more quickly and, depending on the teat, in larger quantities. Look for signs of gulping and spluttering when your infant swallows. This indicates that the teat flow is too fast. Switch to a slow-flow teat or replace your current bottle teat with a newborn size and flow rate.

Bottle-fed babies are more prone to ear infections. As you begin to wean from breast to bottle, feed formula or expressed milk mid-evening and water before bedtime. Milk that collects in the Eustachian tubes is a perfect host for bacteria that can lead to painful ear infections.

Many babies experience nipple/teat confusion when making the transition from breast to bottle. Often they'll refuse to take a bottle from their mother – although the milk tastes and smells the same, the containers are different.

Transition from the breast is a perfect opportunity for Dad to begin feeding his baby. Ask him to offer milk or formula in a bottle or a cup.

Weaning from the Bottle

Weaning from the bottle usually happens somewhere between nine months and two years of age. Older infants and toddlers are often reluctant to give up the bottle because it soothes them to sleep and provides a 'safety zone' at times of anxiety in a big and busy world.

Some parents use the water technique to wean from the bottle. Water is substituted for milk at bedtimes and naptimes, when busy babies and young toddlers seem to want the bottle most often. Because water is less attractive, babies give it up more quickly. If you plan to use this technique, expect some initial resistance. As with all parenting decisions, choose your battles wisely and be consistent once a rule is established.

Keep some perspective on the use of the bottle as a method of feeding your infant. Make yourself, and not the bottle, available to him for physical and emotional comfort throughout the day.

Natural Weaning

Natural weaning is a child-driven process that happens in baby steps usually between the ages of 12 months and three years. When you allow your toddler to set the rhythm, weaning happens naturally. Your hormone levels decline more slowly, and there is little risk of baby blues or breast engorgement. A child's readiness to wean brings closure to the breastfeeding experience. When he initiates the process at his own pace, there are fewer power struggles: it allows him to have a greater sense of control and nurtures his self-esteem.

 Did you know that some mothers can still express breastmilk long after they've weaned their babies or toddlers? In fact, some mothers still have small amounts of milk for up to two or more years following the weaning of their baby. It is not unusual and not a cause for alarm.

Mobile infants and toddlers are easily distracted by outside stimuli and will often wean themselves as they become more independent. While it's important to encourage your child's independence, it's equally important to meet his emotional needs. This is the 'Don't offer, don't refuse' stage of weaning. If your toddler requests to nurse, you can allow it as often and for as long as you wish. But if you don't offer, your busy toddler will find other diversions.

Other Bonding Activities

As they make the transition from the breast, babies still need to be close to their loving parents, both physically and emotionally. Let your baby know you're available to him in other ways besides breastfeeding. He needs the comfort of his mother's arms and plenty of time to cuddle.

Here are a few activities that will continue your nurturing relationship. (In fact, you may find that these activities are good for all nurturing relationships!)

· Colour or draw together
· Cuddle

- Dance
- Do finger plays
- Go on a field trip
- Laugh at funny faces
- Listen to music
- Offer massage
- Read or tell stories to each other
- Recite nursery rhymes
- Rock in a chair
- Sing songs
- Tickle each other.

Breastfeeding gave your child the most natural and healthy start to his or her life, but that was only the beginning. You'll spend the rest of your life concerned with the health and welfare of your children as they continue to grow, learn and become more independent every day. Through all the challenges that come with raising a family, have faith in yourself and your abilities, and remember, above all, to be loving and patient.

Frequently Asked Questions

The information provided in the following pages is addressed in greater detail within the body of this book. FAQs provide an excellent review of breastfeeding in general, and may highlight some of your specific concerns. If you or your baby have special needs, talk to your doctor or health visitor. These professionals can offer you the best advice, based on your personal situation.

Q: **My breasts are small. Can I still breastfeed?**

A: Breast size is not an indicator of your ability to produce milk. However, if you've had breast reduction surgery or have undeveloped breast tissue, talk to your doctor.

Q: **Will it hurt?**

A: Breastfeeding will help relieve the pain of engorgement, which will happen whether you breastfeed or not. There may be some very mild discomfort during the first week while your baby is learning to latch on properly, but it is temporary and not painful.

Q: **My family wants a chance to feed the baby from a bottle. What should I do?**

A: It's important that your baby breastfeeds exclusively for the first six weeks to ensure strong milk production and to avoid nipple/teat confusion. Encourage your family to bond with your baby in other ways, such as bathing, snuggling, rocking and infant massage.

Q: **Can I breastfeed if my nipples are pierced and/or I have breast tattoos?**

A: Most women with pierced nipples can breastfeed without problems, but you should remove your jewellery first. Pierced nipples also tend to leak. Tattoo dyes do not penetrate into the milk-producing cells.

Q: **Why should I breastfeed?**

A: Human milk has been perfected over millions of years of evolution for babies. It is a vital part of a baby's immunity against disease and is easier to digest than other animal milk or artificial formula. Also, breastfeeding provides a woman with some degree of protection against breast cancer. Breastfeeding is nutritious, emotionally satisfying and economical.

Q: **Will breastfeeding make my breasts sag?**

A: No, heredity, pregnancy and age cause breasts to sag.

Q: **How can I breastfeed and go back to work?**

A: Many women continue nursing their babies after they return to work. Some cluster feed at night and express their milk during the day. Employers are increasingly accommodating the needs of nursing mothers.

Talk to your employer about creating a breastfeeding-friendly environment in your workplace.

Q: How can I tell if my baby is getting enough milk?

A: The two best indicators of adequate milk consumption are your baby's weight gain and elimination patterns. If your baby is gaining weight consistently and has between five and eight wet nappies and two to five stools per day (after the first week of life), you are producing enough milk to nourish your baby.

Q: Doesn't breastfeeding tie you down?

A: One of the advantages of breastfeeding is mobility. You can breastfeed anywhere, and with the use of a sling, no one even knows you're doing it.

Q: How often should I feed my baby?

A: During the first week of his life, you will wake your sleepy baby to nurse every two to three hours. Subsequently, your baby will let you know when he's hungry. Babies typically eat eight to 12 times in a 24-hour period.

Q: How can I tell if my baby is hungry?

A: Babies signal hunger by rooting (turning their mouths towards whatever touches their cheek), chewing on their fist and making sounds. Crying is a late hunger cue. You will learn to read your baby's behaviour quickly.

Q: My newborn seems to nurse all the time. Is that normal?

A: Most newborns spend an average of 187 minutes per day nursing during their first two weeks of life. It seems like a lot because they are on the breast every two to three hours, but each session lasts only 15–30 minutes. Babies also tend to nurse more during growth spurts, which happen at around three weeks, six weeks, three months and six months. If your baby nurses often but doesn't wet five to eight nappies per day and have a stool at least two to five times in 24 hours, contact your doctor. This could be an indicator of poor milk consumption.

Q: What if I fall ill and have to take medication?

A: Most medications are compatible with breastfeeding, although many doctors routinely advise temporary weaning. Talk to your GP or health visitor about breastfeeding-friendly medications, as they will be well informed on breastfeeding issues.

Q: Do I have to drink milk to make milk?

A: No. Cows don't, and neither do humans.

Q: Do I have to change my diet to breastfeed?

A: Nursing mothers actually get to eat more than usual. Sometimes certain foods may cause a change in your breastmilk that upsets your baby.

Q: Will exercise make my breastmilk taste bad?

A: Ordinary exercise has not been shown to have any effect on the taste of breastmilk. However, extremely strenuous and prolonged exercise can cause a build-up of lactic acid in breastmilk, which affects the taste for about an hour.

Q: Is it healthy for my older children to watch me nurse my baby?

A: Breastfeeding is a wonderful opportunity to demonstrate breasts functioning the way nature intended. It's also the perfect time to lay the groundwork for sexual education at an age-appropriate level. Children who are raised in breastfeeding homes have a more balanced attitude regarding the human body.

Q: Is it psychologically harmful to breastfeed my toddler?

A: The benefits of breastfeeding continue as long as you nurse your child. Globally, the average age of weaning is three years. Every major health organization recognizes breastfeeding as a healthy and natural means of nurturing children of any age.

Q: Should my baby have cereal to help her sleep through the night?

A: Before six months of age, infants are unable to digest cereal. Not only will cereal upset their stomachs, but it can also cause food allergies.

Q: Isn't nursing in public a form of indecent exposure? Can I be arrested?

A: No one in the UK has ever been convicted of indecent exposure for nursing in public. You have a well-established right to nurse your child anywhere you have the right to be.

Glossary of
Breastfeeding Terms

allergen: A microscopic particle of a substance that can cause an allergic reaction in someone whose immune system is sensitized.

alveoli: Small grape-like clusters of cells in the breast where milk is produced.

amenorrhoea: A term for the halting of the menstrual cycle.

anaesthesia: A drug administered to block pain.

antibodies: Cells in the body that fight foreign cells (e.g. bacteria, fungi and viruses).

areola: The circle of dark breast tissue surrounding the nipple.

aromatherapy: The use of scented oils, candles or other items to influence a person's mental state.

attachment/bonding: The process of forming a strong emotional connection with another person.

baby blues: The short-term feeling of sadness resulting from hormonal imbalance and stress immediately following birth or abrupt weaning from the breast.

babywearing: The practice of carrying an infant on your body, usually in a sling.

bilirubin: A by-product of the breakdown of excess red blood cells. Extremely high levels can cause brain damage.

birth plan: An outline of your desired birthing experience.

breast abscess: An infection of the breast marked by pain, swelling and pus.

breastfeeding: The natural act of feeding a child human milk from the mother's breasts.

breastfeeding counsellor: A professional specializing in the breast and breastfeeding.

breast lobes: The 15–25 internal divisions of the breast, like the sections of an orange.

breast lobules: The 20–40 divisions of each breast lobe that contain milk-producing cells.

breast pump: A mechanical device for expression of breastmilk.

breast shells: Domelike plastic rings used to evert nipples.

Caesarean section: Birthing in which the infant is removed surgically through the mother's abdomen.

candida: See thrush.

casein: The protein in milk that forms hard cottage cheese-like curds in the stomach.

cholecystokinin (CCK): A hormone released from the lining of the stomach that induces a feeling of satisfaction in the brain.

cleft lip/cleft palate: A condition in which an infant's lips do not grow together completely in the womb. Cleft palate refers to a similar condition affecting the roof of a child's mouth.

clogged duct: A condition in which a milk duct becomes clogged, resulting in a hard spot in the breast with accompanying tenderness.

cluster or bunch feeding: Frequent, eager nursings with little time between sessions.

cobedding: The centuries-old practice of sleeping with your baby. Also called the family bed.

colic: A catchall term used to describe any number of conditions in babies whose symptoms include crying continuously for three or more hours, three or more times per week, for three or more weeks.

colostrum: Supermilk produced by mothers in the first few days after birthing.

demand feeding: The practice of breastfeeding a baby when she's hungry, as opposed to a predetermined schedule.

diastasis: A condition in which the vertical abdominal muscles separate during labour.

docosahexaenoic acid (DHA): An important fat that helps build brain tissue in babies.

doll-eye manoeuvre: Bringing your baby to an upright position so that her eyes will open, like the sleep eyes of toy dolls.

double pumping: Using a specially fitted breast pump to express milk from both breasts simultaneously.

doula: A professional labour assistant.

eczema: A skin condition characterized by dry, patchy skin.

engorgement: The enlargement of a woman's breasts caused by the onset of milk production or the build-up of milk following abrupt weaning.

evert: To make protrude; the opposite of invert.

exclusive breastfeeding: The practice of feeding a baby nothing but breastmilk.

extended nursing: Breastfeeding children who are beyond one year of age.

family bed: See cobedding.

finger feeding: Allowing an infant to suckle on a clean adult finger while breastmilk is introduced into the mouth through a syringe or supplemental feeding tube.

flow rate: The speed at which milk flows through a bottle teat.

foremilk: The first milk baby receives during a nursing session. Foremilk is low in fat and high in volume.

frenulum: The thin strip of tissue that connects the bottom of the tongue to the floor of the mouth.

galactose: One of the two sugars formed by the digestion of lactose.

galactosaemia: A hereditary condition in which a child cannot digest galactose.

gastro-oesophageal reflux (GER): A condition in which the muscular valve at the juncture of the stomach and throat allows stomach contents and acid into the oesophagus, causing a painful, heartburn-like sensation.

gavage: Feeding method in which a tube is inserted through a baby's mouth and into the stomach.

glucose: A simple sugar.

hindmilk: The breastmilk released after several minutes of nursing. Hindmilk is rich in fat and important nutrients.

hunger cues: Signals that a baby is hungry. These typically include rooting, chewing on a fist and crying.

hypoglycaemia: Low blood sugar.

hypothalamus: A part of the brain that regulates many autonomic functions such as body temperature and milk production.

hypothyroidism: A condition in which the thyroid gland is underactive, resulting in many symptoms, including a diminished milk supply.

immune system: The body's protection against disease.

infant formula: Any of the artificial liquid foods designed for babies. Infant formulas are usually based on animal milk or soya.

inverted nipples: Nipples that do not protrude from the breast when stimulated.

involute: The process by which the uterus contracts following childbirth, returning to its pre-pregnancy size.

jaundice: A typical condition of newborns in which the child is excessively sleepy and exhibits yellowing of her skin and the whites of her eyes. Jaundice is caused by an excess of red blood cells.

kangaroo care: A style of newborn care used successfully for premature infants. The baby is placed on the mother's chest with skin-to-skin contact and ready access to the breast.

lactation: The medical term for the production of milk.

lactogenesis: The onset of milk production.

lactose: Milk sugar.

latch: The connection between baby and breast.

letdown reflex: See milk ejection reflex.

lochia: The menses-like flow of blood from the vagina following birth.

lumpectomy: The removal of a growth or tumour without destruction of surrounding tissues.

manual expression: Removing milk from the breast using the hand.

mastectomy: Surgical removal of all or part of the breast.

mastitis: An infection of the breast characterized by flu-like symptoms and swelling, redness and tenderness of the affected breast.

mature milk: Breastmilk produced after five days post partum.

meconium: Greenish-black, tar-like stool present in newborns.

milk bank: Storage, preparation and distribution facilities for donated human milk.

milk ducts: The channels connecting the alveoli to the milk sinuses.

milk ejection reflex: The release of breastmilk from the milk-producing cells of the breast, caused by muscular contractions in response to oxytocin.

milk sinuses: The area beneath the areola that must be compressed to force milk through the nipple.

Montgomery glands: The small bumps on the areolae of a lactating woman that produce a substance that keeps the nipples clean and lubricated.

mylenization: The covering of nerve fibres with an insulating layer of fat.

neonatal intensive care unit (NICU): Intensive care unit for newborns such as premature infants, or others suffering from neonatal illnesses, diseases or disorders.

nipple shields: Thin plastic protectors that fit over a mother's nipples as she nurses her child.

nursing strike: A baby's abrupt refusal to breastfeed due to some interfering factor such as teething pain, a blocked nose or even Mum's new perfume.

oestrogen: The primary female sex hormone; produced mainly in the ovaries.

orthodontic teats: Bottle teats that are designed to help a baby's oral cavity and teeth develop properly.

oxytocin: The hormone responsible for the milk ejection reflex.

pelvic floor exercise: An exercise for tightening and strengthening the muscles of the perineal floor.

perineum: The connective tissue between the vagina and the anus.

phenylalanine: An important amino acid.

phenylketonuria (PKU): An inherited disorder in which the body is unable to properly utilize phenylalanine.

phototherapy: The use of special lights in the treatment of newborn jaundice and seasonal affective disorder.

pituitary gland: The body's master gland, which produces many hormones, including prolactin and oxytocin.

post partum: Following labour and delivery.

postnatal depression (PND): Feelings of despair or hopelessness following the birth of a baby and lasting longer than two weeks.

postnatal psychosis: A rare disorder of mothers characterized by hallucinations, delusions and extreme confusion.

premature infant: A child born before 36 weeks' gestation.

preterm milk: Breastmilk produced by the mother of a premature infant. Preterm milk is especially high in fats, proteins and sugars.

progesterone: Along with oestrogen, progesterone is one of the two primary female hormones regulating fertility.

progestin: The synthetic version of progesterone.

prolactin: The hormone responsible for milk production.

relactating: Re-establishing breastmilk production after it has been stopped.

seasonal affective disorder (SAD): A physiological condition of depression caused by a lack of sunlight and activity. SAD is most common in northern latitudes.

sleep apnoea: A condition in which a person stops breathing during sleep, often occurring many times throughout the night and requiring the sufferer to wake in order to begin breathing again.

sleep/wake cycle: The states of consciousness and arousability. They include: quiet alert, active alert, crying, drowsiness, active sleep and deep sleep.

sudden infant death syndrome (SIDS): Also called cot death.

supplemental feeding: Feeding done in addition to or in place of breastfeeding.

swaddling: Wrapping a baby snugly in a blanket. The practice of swaddling helps a young infant to feel secure and warm.

tandem nursing: Breastfeeding more than one child.

thrush: A yeast infection of a baby's mouth and, subsequently, the mother's nipples.

tongue thrust: The reflexive ejection of anything placed in a baby's mouth.

transitional milk: The mix of colostrum and mature milk.

weaning: The process of transitioning a child away from the breast.

wet nurse: A woman who is paid to breastfeed a child other than her own.

yeast infection: Any infection caused by yeast fungi. See thrush.

Index

Page numbers in **bold** refer to illustrations.